A Life in Academic Medicine

A Life in Academic Medicine

Philip J. Snodgrass, M.D.
Professor of Medicine Emeritus
Indiana University School of
Medicine

iUniverse, Inc.
New York Lincoln Shanghai

A Life in Academic Medicine

Copyright © 2007 by Philip J. Snodgrass

All rights reserved. No part of this book may be used or reproduced by any means, graphic, electronic, or mechanical, including photocopying, recording, taping or by any information storage retrieval system without the written permission of the publisher except in the case of brief quotations embodied in critical articles and reviews.

iUniverse books may be ordered through booksellers or by contacting:

iUniverse
2021 Pine Lake Road, Suite 100
Lincoln, NE 68512
www.iuniverse.com
1-800-Authors (1-800-288-4677)

Because of the dynamic nature of the Internet, any Web addresses or links contained in this book may have changed since publication and may no longer be valid.

The views expressed in this work are solely those of the author and do not necessarily reflect the views of the publisher, and the publisher hereby disclaims any responsibility for them.

ISBN: 978-0-595-44253-9 (pbk)
ISBN: 978-0-595-88584-8 (ebk)

Printed in the United States of America

Dedicated to my wife, Marjorie, for her loving support and wise counsel, and to my many teachers and colleagues during my life in medicine.

Contents

Preface ix

Chapter 1   What Led Me to Medicine 1

Chapter 2   Harvard Medical School 7

Chapter 3   Internship 29
Peter Bent Brigham Hospital, 1953–1954

Chapter 4   U.S. Navy Medical Reserve 43
Kingsville, Texas, 1954–1956

Chapter 5   Junior Residency 56
Peter Bent Brigham Hospital, 1956–1957

Chapter 6   Research Training 67
Biophysics Research Laboratory, 1957–1959

Chapter 7   Senior Residency 73
Peter Bent Brigham Hospital, 1959–1960

Chapter 8   Chief Residency 80
Peter Bent Brigham Hospital, 1961–1963

Chapter 9   Chief of Gastroenterology 90
Peter Bent Brigham Hospital, 1963–1968

Chapter 10   Chief of Gastroenterology 109
Peter Bent Brigham Hospital, 1969–1973

Chapter 11   Chief of the VA Medical Service and Professor of Medicine 117
Indiana University School of Medicine, 1973–1981

CHAPTER 12   Sabbatical Leave.......................... 133
    Oxford, England, 1982

CHAPTER 13   Chief of the VA Medical Service and Professor of
             Medicine 139
    Indiana University School of Medicine, 1983–1995

CHAPTER 14   Retirement............................... 147

Index... 155

Preface

ooooooooooooooooooooooooooooooo
"Life is not what one lived, but what one remembers, and how one remembers it in order to recount it."

—*Gabriel García Márquez*

Why another memoir by a medical doctor? Is there anything that I can add that is new, unique or of historical interest to the other books of this kind? My viewpoint is that following World War Two there began a golden period during which medical care and biomedical research blossomed, in great part because of government support through the National Institutes of Health. I was fortunate to begin Harvard Medical School in 1949, where major advances in health care and research were being made. Again, by good fortune, I was accepted for training at the Peter Bent Brigham Hospital, which was a Harvard teaching hospital and though small was the site of major advances in care and research. Thus the experiences that I relate in this memoir are a reflection of U.S. medicine from the 1940s through the 1990s.

What is **academic** medicine? It is a special career niche among the wide spectrum of careers in medical practice and science. The key features are that academic medicine exists primarily to teach medical students and to train doctors after medical school. In common with many university professors, medical school professors also do research and their promotions rely primarily on the publication of their research efforts. The greatest contrast with other academics is that professors of medicine also take care of sick people. Thus they are expected to be "triple threat" doctors, skilled at teaching, up-to-date and even leaders in their field of research and competent if not excellent in their area of patient care. This tripod upon which academic medicine sits was the academic ideal taught us at Harvard and the Brigham. Achieving excellence in research and patient care became ever more difficult as knowledge proliferated in all three areas during the latter half of the twentieth century. This memoir is the story of one person's attempt to accomplish all three requirements of academic medicine, including his successes and failures.

I chose to present this story in a reportorial style, avoiding opinions and commentary where possible. I tried not to lead the readers toward my conclusions about this challenging life's work. The facts should lead the readers to their own conclusions. As many will realize, success is now possible in basic science research mostly by MDs with an additional PhD degree or in a laboratory staffed with a group of PhDs. Basic research MDs can teach medical students in their basic science courses but they rarely can continue with patient care. In clinical research it is still possible to combine this activity with patient care and teaching. Many academic doctors now do only patient care and some teaching.

My memoir thus depicts the efforts of a specialist in internal medicine, gastroenterology and liver disease and also a biochemist to create a career in academic medicine. Doctors who are surgeons, neurologists or psychiatrists and attempt to do academic medicine face their own special challenges. Any young person planning a career in medicine may profit from the lessons learned by me and my colleagues over the past 50 years.

I have chosen to identify major figures in my life by name and have recounted my interactions with them as truthfully as my memory allowed me to do so. Readers who knew them may differ from me in their memories or opinions about them. All omissions or misinterpretations in this memoir rest entirely with the author.

1

What Led Me to Medicine

Beginning in junior high school, I had the vague idea that I wanted to become a doctor. There was no particular reason for this. My father was a lawyer, not a doctor. I had an uncle who was a surgeon, but I didn't know him very well and cannot honestly say that he was a role model. My family doctor was an internist whom I liked and respected, but again I did not think of him as my role model. I read some books about physicians, mostly fiction, but none of them took me by storm. However, during the summer between 10th and 11th grade in high school in Madison, Wisconsin, I decided to test out whether I might like a life in medicine. I obtained a job as an orderly at Wisconsin General Hospital, which is the large teaching hospital at the University of Wisconsin School of Medicine. I was paid the enormous sum of $0.35 an hour to work a 48-hour week. I was assigned to a general surgical ward where there were forty patients going to and coming back from all kinds of surgery; chest, abdominal, head and neck, burns, and cancer surgery. This was during World War II and most of the doctors and nurses were in the armed forces. Our busy ward was staffed with one head-nurse, one or two student nurses and me. In those days there were no nurse's aides or licensed practical nurses. The patients were divided up in the morning to receive their bed-baths, a change of their bed linen, a shave, and any other treatments they needed including enemas. I became quite paranoid about the fact that I always seemed to be assigned to the most soiled patients. One of these was a dying elderly man who had cancer of the rectum and was incontinent of feces. When I arrived in the morning, he would be covered with feces from head to toe, requiring an enormous clean-up procedure. I continued to care for him until he died. We also had a man with a 50 percent burn, who every day was placed in a huge old-fashioned bathtub with some kind of salt solution, probably Epsom salts, to soak his infected burns and clean up his wounds. My painful memory was that the tub was full of blood every time we gave him his bath. Another of my patients had cancer in his throat, which had eaten through into his neck tissue so that it was open and infected and had a terrible, foul odor. I was quite astounded when they placed maggots in the wound to clean up the necrotic material and it worked. This poor man paced the floor moaning in pain in spite of narcotics and finally was released from his misery by death.

I also ended up being the ward errand boy, taking people in wheelchairs or on carts around the hospital for various treatments. One of my amusing memories is that I had to shave many of these old men with a safety razor and I did a terrible job of it. One of them pointed out that I didn't have enough beard, at the age of 15, to require shaving myself daily yet, which was true. My best friend, Eugene Dye, also was interested in medicine and had a job at Wisconsin General Hospital that summer. He was assigned to the psychiatric ward and I visited him at regular intervals. There I saw the results of a procedure called a frontal lobotomy, in which a hole was made on both sides of the front of the skull and a knife was pushed through the frontal lobes to separate them from the rest of the brain. I saw one man, formerly a salesman, who prior to the procedure was driven by a manic urge to sell, interrupted by episodes of depression leading to multiple suicide attempts. After this frontal lobotomy procedure, he became a man with no personality and no initiative, but at least he quit attempting suicide.

I do not remember much about the interns and residents or the professors. If they came on the ward, I was too busy to follow them around and I never got to know them. Near the end of August, I became quite ill with a high fever and was admitted to the medical ward at Wisconsin General Hospital. I think they feared that I had picked up some illness working there. My rectal temperature, according to what I was told later, gradually rose to 108 degrees Fahrenheit, almost always a lethal level. Before I lapsed into a coma, I remember my mother sitting at my bedside sponging my face with cool cloths and saying "Philip, you are not going to die. Philip, you are not going to die." The Chief of Medicine at Wisconsin General, Ovid Meyer, was my doctor and I know that he did everything he could, including giving me an intravenous sulfa drug on the theory that I had some bacterial infection. I recovered in a week without major complications. When I went back to work for the final two weeks of the summer, I went into the record room and looked into my hospital chart to see what diagnosis I was given. They signed me out as "summer disease," question viral infection. Apparently these were the limits of science at that time. Looking back on this summer's experience, I wonder why I still wanted to become a doctor.

Nevertheless the next summer, between my junior and senior years in high school, I signed up again to be a hospital orderly. This time, I went to a small private hospital in Madison because I thought I would get to know people better. I was assigned to a mixed medical and surgical ward. I recall that we had only one intern and no resident physicians. This hospital did not get interns every year and was not considered a good choice by those who graduated from the medical school at Wisconsin. If the intern or staff physician wanted to find out why a patient died, he would obtain permission for an autopsy and the intern had to assist with the autopsy. For example, I recall a 60-year-old farmer who developed abdominal pain while making hay in August. At the end of a long workday he felt so sick that he went to see his doctor, who diagnosed him as probable appendicitis and sent him into our hospital. He was very ill when he arrived and went immediately to surgery. I remember "scrubbing in" so I could watch the procedure and maybe lend a pair of hands. When they opened his abdomen, he had infection everywhere, generalized peritonitis due to a ruptured appendix. The surgeon took out his appendix, irrigated the abdominal cavity with saline and then sprinkled sulfa powder throughout his abdomen, as you would sprinkle salt from a shaker. Amazingly, this tough old farmer survived the surgery and at the end of a week he looked like he was about to recover. I helped him to the bathroom, his first trip there on his own, and on our way back to the bed, he suddenly collapsed and we could not resuscitate him. The intern and I were very sad because of the death of this brave man. The intern requested and got permission to do an autopsy. I went to the morgue and watched him open up the man's chest and remove the heart and lungs. He found huge blood clots (thrombi) in the main pulmonary artery and in the branches of the pulmonary artery. Some of the clot was still coiled up in the right ventricle. He had developed blood clots in his leg veins after the surgery and during bed rest. The clots broke loose when he first got up, walked and strained to have his first bowel movement. This memory stayed with me throughout my later medical career and I always struggled to prevent these tragic deaths by pulmonary embolism.

The intern also assisted in the delivery room and he told me a most disturbing story about a delivery he witnessed. A general practitioner who had privileges to deliver babies got into trouble. The baby got caught high up in the birth canal, so-called high transverse arrest. He did not know how do a high forceps delivery and did not call for help. He reached up into the womb and broke up the baby manually and pulled it out in pieces. He told the mother afterwards that her baby had been stillborn and never allowed her to see the child. I urged the intern to report this disaster to the hospital director but he was afraid that he would be discharged as a troublemaker. I heard from the intern that this doctor had a reputation for bad outcomes of his obstetrical cases. There was no investigation of this baby's death. This doctor was never told that he could no longer do obstetrics.

When I graduated from high school in June of 1945, I was only 17 years old, turning 18 on November 3rd. The war was still going on with Japan and I knew that I was due for induction into the armed forces. Stimulated by the guidance counselor at my high school, a wonderful maiden lady, I applied to Harvard College and to my astonishment I was admitted along with my best friend, Eugene Dye, and another boy from our class. At that time it was easier to get into Harvard College than it is now. Because of the army looming in the future, we decided at least to get in a summer term, so we took the train to Boston and started after the Fourth of July for an eight-week summer semester. While in Cambridge, I had to go to the post office for my army physical. In spite of a height of 6 feet and a weight of 115 pounds, I passed and was ordered to report for induction in early September at Fort Sheridan, Illinois. In mid-August, President Truman ordered the dropping of the bombs on Hiroshima and Nagasaki and the Japanese surrendered. I joined other Harvard students who went downtown in Boston to celebrate VJ Day. We jumped on a fire engine and rode all over the North End of Boston while people threw strands of toilet paper out the windows as confetti. When school was finished I flew home because I still had that notice to report for induction. When I arrived home another notification came through that President Truman had canceled the draft and no more inductions would occur.

I have looked back on these events many times and have concluded that I am probably alive today because I did not have to go and fight in the invasion of Japan. The use of the two atomic bombs, in my personal opinion, was necessary to convince the Japanese to end the war. I have seen estimates from both Japanese and U.S. archives that the deaths of both Americans and Japanese would have been around 12 million if we had had to fight our way through the islands.

Back at Harvard College for the fall term I learned that my freshman advisor, a famous archeologist, was off in the Yucatan on a dig. Therefore I had to see the freshman Dean for counseling about my choice of courses and my eventual area of concentration. I told him that I wanted to apply to medical school when I finished college. He looked a bit irritated because he had probably heard this from too many college freshmen. He pointed out that my College Board test scores were high in everything but math and chemistry and that I had excelled in European history in the summer term. He said that I should consider a different career from medicine, something derived from the humanities. I did not take his advice but registered my concentration as biochemistry.

During the summer term, I was required to take English Composition, which after some difficulties I finally brought up to an A grade. I also began European history and was one of two students who received an A. I had to take trigonometry, logarithms, analytical geometry and introduction to calculus, because I hadn't taken these in high school. I only received a B. In the fall term, I finished European history and started a double German course, receiving A grades in both, but in differential calculus and inorganic chemistry received Bs. To my great surprise these grades earned me the Detur Award, given to the eight students with the best academic records in the first year of college. I achieved this record by being what my friends called a "greasy grind," not because I was smarter than any of them. Fortunately for me I discovered rowing, which gave me a needed respite from studying. I rowed three years on the lightweight crew, never rising higher than the junior varsity, and learned to row a single shell in my senior year. I loved rowing so much that I have continued to row a single all my life, competing in races all over the U.S.

In my sophomore year I excelled in the humanities and struggled in the sciences. The Dean's predictions were becoming true. This made me reconsider whether I shouldn't give up the idea of going to medical school and try to get a PhD in history or literature. My final two years only confirmed these concerns. I enjoyed my science courses even though I had to work much harder to master the material than I did in history, philosophy, literature and music. I did a tutorial in biochemistry with a kind and demanding man named John Edsall, who I learned later was one of the most distinguished American biochemists. I wrote a library research thesis on the synthesis of purines, where I learned about the breakthrough role of radioactive-labeled compounds in intermediary metabolism. In February 1949 I graduated from Harvard College cum laude, with a major in biochemical sciences. I was still concerned that I was not strong in math, physics and chemistry. Was this a defect that would prevent me from being a good doctor?

During my summer vacations in college I worked on the University of Wisconsin Experimental Farm in the department of horticulture. I earned a good salary as a state civil servant during those summers and this helped me pay for college. As a field hand, I tended test plots of fruits and vegetables, helped develop hybrid corn varieties adapted for each growing season in Wisconsin and assisted a professor who was doing research on weed prevention with the chemical plant hormone 2-4D. I planted vegetables, treated plots set out in Latin (random) squares and counted the numbers of different weed types in each plot. I observed how the results were analyzed statistically. This professor was so successful in his weed control research that he went to Cornell University as a full professor in their department of horticulture.

At the end of my last Fall semester in 1948 at Harvard College I decided to apply to medical schools in spite of my concerns about whether medical science was my best talent.

2

Harvard Medical School

In the late fall of 1948, I applied for admission to medical school at the University of Wisconsin, Harvard and Michigan. I fully expected to attend the University of Wisconsin because it was my home-state school and the cost would be much lower. My family expected that after medical school I would be trained as a surgeon and join the Pember-Nuzum Clinic in Janesville, Wisconsin as an assistant surgeon to my uncle Thomas Snodgrass. The Pember-Nuzum Clinic was founded by Dr. Aubrey Pember, an obstetrician, and my great-uncle, Dr. Thomas Nuzum, a surgeon who continued to operate until he reached the age of 90. Finally the other clinic physicians took away his operating room privileges but allowed him to follow his patients until he died at age 97. His nephew, Dr. Thomas J. Snodgrass, then became the leading partner at the clinic. My cousin, Dr. Herbert Snodgrass, joined the clinic as an internist. Everyone in my extended family hoped that I would become a doctor and join the clinic.

I called for an interview during my winter vacation in Madison and the only person available to see me was Dr. William S. Middleton, the Dean of the school. He looked over my record from Harvard and commented on the fact that I had Cs in organic chemistry, physical chemistry and physics. He pointed out that he could fill all of the positions at Wisconsin with straight-A students and asked why he should take a person with a record like mine. I pointed out that physical chemistry was the toughest course that I took in all of college. It was taught by a Nobel Prize winner, Professor E. B. Wilson, who said that he would not soften the course for premedical students but would expect us to compete with those who were majoring in chemistry. Dean Middleton asked me, "Are you implying that a C at Harvard is equal to an A at Wisconsin?" I said "No, you said that, not I." He said, "You left Wisconsin to go to college out East and therefore you are not really an in-state applicant." I pointed out that my father's family pioneered in Wisconsin in 1850 and that many of my family members had attended the University of Wisconsin. I pointed that he was the outsider because he came to

Wisconsin from Pennsylvania. After this unpleasant interaction he said that he would not admit me to the University of Wisconsin Medical School.

When I got back to Boston, I received a telephone call from Harvard Medical School asking me if I could come over that morning for an interview with a Dr. Kendall Emerson at the Peter Bent Brigham Hospital. Naturally I hastened over and we had a pleasant discussion. We talked about my experience rowing on the lightweight junior varsity crew, which he thought was a fine activity. He asked me one scientific question: "Recently a metal has been found at the center of vitamin B12. Do you know about that?" Luckily, I had read one of the recent editions of *Nature* and knew that it was cobalt. He was impressed enough to say, "I think you deserve to be admitted to this school." So I received my acceptance in January to enter Harvard Medical School in September 1949.

I moved to Beacon Hill with a friend from Kirkland House at Harvard. We shared a room in the five-story row house of Mrs. Augustus Lowell Putnam at 84 Revere St. She was a brilliant and handsome woman who had been involved in a famous scandal. As a result, Lucy Putnam was banned from polite society, but found a fascinating group of friends who were writers and artists. She was very kind to me. One of the things that endeared her to me was that when I had a date, she would allow my friends and me to use her living room to entertain young ladies. They were always impressed by that Beacon Hill house.

During that spring, I obtained a job in the Department of Medicine at Harvard Medical School in the Hematology Research Lab directed by Dr. Clement Finch. He was the chief of hematology at the Peter Bent Brigham Hospital and a renowned expert on hemochromatosis, an iron storage disease. He had working with him a cousin, Stuart Finch, who went on to Yale as a professor of hematology, and another young man, E. Donnall Thomas, who was scheduled to be the chief resident at the Peter Bent Brigham Hospital the next year. Dr. Thomas went on to win the Nobel Prize in Medicine for successfully pioneering bone marrow transplants. My job was to set up a new method to analyze iron in tissues. I went to the chemistry library at Harvard College, looked at a number of methods and finally chose one which turned out to be tedious and probably inaccurate. I did not consult with experts in iron analysis at the college or the medical school. I was an example of the overweening self-confidence of a new graduate from Harvard College. Clem Finch and I had a number of arguments about my work. The research in Finch's lab was done helter-skelter. I could not see any clear hypotheses and I was not impressed by what was he called clinical research. He thought I was a "wise guy" and he was correct. I told him that he was an artist in "slinging the bull." Luckily for me he went to the new medical school at the

University of Washington in Seattle as chief of hematology. I never asked him for a recommendation!

I found some interesting friends in Building D, where our lab was located. One was Dr. Harold Amos, a research fellow who became one of the first black full professors at Harvard Medical School and later chairman of the Department of Bacteriology and Immunology. Another young PhD lived on Beacon Hill and we commuted together. He was trying to isolate the beta-streptococcal antigens that caused rheumatic fever, but purification methods in those days were too primitive for him to succeed.

I began medical school in September and on the first day as I entered the dining room to eat lunch I saw my Harvard College acquaintances in one corner of the room. Harvard supplied 30 members of the class of 100. I looked around and saw another table with three strangers. I wanted to get to know other people in the class so I sat down and introduced myself. This is how I met Geoffrey Coley from Yale, Frederik Hansen from the College of Puget Sound, and John Whitcomb from Oberlin. We hit it off so well at lunch and thereafter that we decided to become a four-person anatomy dissection team. This decision to seek new friends changed my life in medical school. Our class was full of outstanding people. Among them, David Gray from Princeton, John Sacci from West Virginia, and Norman Crisp from Dartmouth became close friends of mine. I also kept up with most of my Harvard College classmates, particularly Dan Federman, who later became the president of our class; John Mannick, who went on to be the chief of surgery at the Peter Bent Brigham; Chris Martin, who was later chief of medical affairs at Merck laboratories; and Don Louria, who became a professor of preventive medicine at the Medical College of New Jersey.

The first year was truly a grind. Gross anatomy in those days was not functional anatomy, but required masses of memorization without any idea of what that wonderful anatomy was designed to accomplish. Our histology course was taught by Professor Don Fawcett and colleagues. Don was one of the pioneers in electron microscopy of tissues and a great teacher. In the Second Year Show I was privileged to "take him off." I had a wonderful partner in histology, but lost him at the end of the first year. He went home for the summer vacation and died of a ruptured cerebral aneurysm. The biochemistry course was a great disappointment. There were some excellent professors but others were disappointing. My course in biochemistry at Harvard College was much better. The physiology course was outstanding and ahead of its time. I made a life-long friend of Abraham Clifford Barger, who was my instructor in cardiac and pulmonary physiology. The best thing about physiology was that they taught not just masses of information, but principles that served me in good stead the rest of my life. One of the weaknesses of the curriculum in those days was the lack of practical experience with patients. We rarely saw patients, and then only in demonstration clinics. We felt unconnected to the practice of medicine. In an attempt to see something clinical, I asked a gynecologist-obstetrician at the Boston Lying-In Hospital to let me scrub in while he delivered a baby. The young woman who was having her first child was put under general anesthesia and when the baby was delivered it was anencephalic, that is, the brain had never developed except for the brain stem. The baby was put aside and allowed to die because it did not breathe spontaneously. The mother was never shown the child but told that her baby was stillborn. I was horrified by this tragedy.

My first year was academically disappointing. I thought that medical school required too much memorizing and that it was not scholarly in the way postgraduate studies in the liberal arts were. I began to go to the library on my own and read about clinically relevant topics. I read in depth about hypertension which at that time had no effective treatment. My stress level was quite high. We had frequent tests and if we did not pass them, we received a pink slip in our mailbox. In an attempt to deal with the stress, I continued to exercise as I had in college, but I could not find time to go to the Harvard boathouse and continue rowing a single shell, which I learned to do in my last semester of college. I took up squash, which gives aerobic exercise in a short period of time. I worked on the various boxing bags, a carryover from my boxing experience in college. An immature approach to stress reduction by some of us was drinking parties. I went along with some of the first-year students as we made fools of ourselves getting drunk at fraternity and other social occasions. Strangely, I never did this in college.

Every Friday night after the weekly quizzes, some of us would decompress by having parties in our rooms in Vanderbilt Hall. We would invite attractive young women, feed them alcoholic beverages and some would try to get them to go to bed. For personal reasons, I never tried seriously to accomplish the final goal. The Longwood medical area was surrounded by women's colleges and nursing schools and there was no shortage of willing and attractive young women, many of whom ended up marrying medical students. I had remained a virgin all through high school and college and I remained so in medical school despite the temptations. My reasons for doing this were not all high-minded. I was afraid of getting a girl pregnant or contracting a venereal disease. Fundamentally, I was trying to live up to my parents' and family's expectations about my behavior. I dated many interesting and attractive girls during my first year but not seriously. I kept up a more serious relationship with a girl from Smith College whom I met in my freshman year in college. Marriage was something I considered only after graduation from medical school.

One of my best friends, John Whitcomb, lived next door to me on the fifth floor. He was engaged to a young woman named Dorothy Bradley, whom he had met at Oberlin College where he attended for three years. He told me of a summer that he spent in the U.S Forest Service in Idaho while he was in college. It sounded idyllic. I needed a break from studying in medical school, so I applied for and was accepted as a worker on a crew fighting the white pine blister rust (a fungus) in the Clearwater National Forest in Idaho. Its headquarters was in Pierce, Idaho, the old gold-mining capitol, at 7000 feet altitude, near the Lolo Trail followed by Lewis and Clark. One of my friends in medical school, Jim Peters from Princeton, also agreed to work with me in the Forest Service.

I visited my cousin and his family in Minneapolis and then boarded the Great Northern train, the Empire Builder, heading for Spokane, Washington. A lady sitting next to me explained that she was going to a funeral with her sister, who was seated in the car ahead. After listening to her talk nonstop for an hour, I gallantly agreed to trade seats so that she could sit with her sister. I carried her sister's suitcase back to our car and took my duffle bag up to the next car. There was a girl sitting behind me next to a rancher and they chatted until he got off in Montana. I stood up and asked if I could sit with her and talk. She said yes, so I sat down and met Marjorie Lagemann, whose nickname from Oberlin College was "Woody." She had just graduated and lived next door in the senior dorm to Dorothy Bradley, who was marrying John Whitcomb that very week. We had each sent a wedding present to them before we left for the West. She was going to a Girl Scout camp on Lake Coeur d'Alene in Idaho and fortunately for me she explained that she was returning to Boston in the fall to go to school and teach at Perkins Institution for the Blind in Watertown, Massachusetts. After talking for ten hours, we got off the train in Spokane and promised to write one another, which I faithfully did and she answered. One night we were able to meet in Lewiston, Idaho on the Snake River, I driving down from the mountains with a friend and she driving from her camp with counselor friends. We spent hours talking in an orchard. Thus began a romance which has persisted throughout my whole life.

The work in the Forest Service blister rust camp consisted of searching thousands of acres in the mountains at eight to ten thousand feet looking for gooseberry bushes and other species of *Ribes*, which were the intermediate host of a fungus, the blister rust, which attacked the white pine, girdled the limbs and killed the trees. This Clearwater Forest was a mature white pine forest worth incredible amounts of money and the Forest Service decided that they had better take care of it until it came time to log it. Every worker at our camp was a forestry major in his university doing a summer internship except for Jim Peters and myself. Jim became famous throughout the Clearwater camps because he would not buy leather, caulked hiking boots like the rest of us but wore white buck shoes all summer. The work consisted of climbing up a thousand feet every morning and spending the day scrambling up and down acres of dense forest, shrubs and rocks, digging out *Ribes* bushes. I enjoyed the experience, gained the best physical condition of my life and came away with a tremendous admiration for the professionals who ran the U.S. Forest Service at that time.

When I got back to Boston, the first thing I did was call Marjorie (Woody) at Perkins. I took her to dinner and we hit it off wonderfully again. We began dating steadily. She finally convinced me to quit the Friday night drinking parties. In order to get to Watertown and back without having to use the slow Boston bus and trolley system, I purchased a 1929 four-door Model A Ford from a Harvard College student and used it to commute to Watertown and later on to the hospitals around Boston. This is the only car I have ever owned that I could take care of myself.

In the second year of medical school I began the year-long course in pathology, general and organ-oriented, a tough but interesting course. I realize now that what I learned in pathology has essentially been the mental model of disease that I have carried in my head ever since. I also took a semester of pharmacology and found myself dealing with Professor Avram Goldstein, a young and brilliant teacher whose lectures and examinations were a great puzzle to me. He gave me my first pink slip, a big blow to my ego. We also took bacteriology, another massive memorization course. Somehow I missed out on the fact that the greatest advances in the new area of molecular biology were occurring in bacteriology

That summer after my second year, I drove with my fiancée, Marjorie Lagemann, to Indianapolis to meet her family and to announce our engagement. I sensed that her family was quite wary of me, coming from Harvard Medical School and a family that they thought was wealthy. We then drove on to Madison to meet my family. My mother welcomed Woody and understood her difficulties trying to meet and please the family of her fiancée, a problem that she had had when she became engaged to my father. She generously offered to pay for the engagement ring, which I could not afford. My father took a hearty dislike to Woody because she was "only a poor school teacher's daughter from Indianapolis." He had hoped that I would marry a rich girl from Boston. My younger sister took the clue from my father and did not warm to Woody. My brother, Richard, who was just then leaving for active duty in the Air Force, had become disillusioned from his first two years at the University of Wisconsin, changing his major almost every semester and uncertain about what to do with his life. So he decided to join the Air Force and he made a career there over the next twenty-two years, rising from enlisted man to bombardier-navigator to B-52 pilot and lieutenant colonel. Although jealous of my success at Harvard and my settled career goal, he welcomed Woody into the family. Woody had obtained a summer job in Madison with the Dane County Girl Scout Council. She worked with scouts in the city and at the camp. After a training period she led four canoes full of girls down the Wisconsin River. Unfortunately, the time they chose was after huge rainstorms had occurred and the Wisconsin River was in flood. A three-day trip lasted one day as they roared along in the flood, dodging chicken coops and other debris. Fortunately she was an experienced counselor and canoeist.

During this summer in Madison I obtained a job at the University of Wisconsin School of Medicine working for a pathologist who had just returned from the war and was doing research on acute renal failure, which was also called acute tubular necrosis. The doctor had served in the army as a general medical officer and found himself in the invasion of Anzio, the beachhead north of Rome, which the Americans thought would cut the Germans off in the middle of the Italian Peninsula. The Americans got caught by superior German forces and suffered huge losses while stuck on that beachhead. My professor, who was more of a scientist than a practicing physician, ended up in the front lines giving emergency triage treatment to wounded soldiers. He saw many soldiers suffer severe shock (low blood pressure) from wounds and loss of blood. Even when they survived the surgery, they often went into acute kidney failure and died of the complications within two or three weeks. When he got back to the medical school at Wisconsin to resume his academic career, he decided to try to work out the pathophysiology of acute tubular necrosis. He found that rabbits were very sensitive to changes in blood pressure and to infusions of various toxic substances that are released when muscles are crushed, such as hemoglobin and myoglobin. He was able to reproduce in these rabbits acute kidney failure by putting them into hemorrhagic shock and then giving them back their blood or by giving them mild shock and then an infusion of myoglobin or hemoglobin or phosphate. Under the microscope the kidney injury closely resembled that seen in humans with acute tubular necrosis.

The professor was ahead of his time and I don't know if he ever got credit for what he found. I guess that he was not good at writing up and publishing his results. I was not a great help in the laboratory. I ruined the ear veins of a lot of rabbits and accidentally killed some rabbits which were struggling in the restraint boxes and broke their own necks. I don't think he considered me a great candidate for a future in research in physiology or biochemistry. I also did a few simple laboratory procedures on urine and blood. My experience with the professor did inspire me that someday I might be able to do research on human disease and figure out the causes of something important. I was impressed by his patience, his careful recording of data, his honesty and his humility. Maybe he was too humble and didn't take credit for what he had accomplished.

After this experience in the summer of 1951, I became officially engaged to Marjorie Lagemann, drove her back to Indianapolis and then went on to Boston for my first clinical experience of medical school. My classmate Scott Earle and I had signed up for a two-week obstetrics rotation in Providence, Rhode Island, at the Providence Lying-In Hospital, which delivered the fourth-highest number of babies in the United States each year. We had heard only a few lectures on pregnancy and delivery and had no practical knowledge. The night we arrived, one of the residents showed us on a model how the baby (a doll) moved through the birth canal and how we should assist the exit. After dinner, we got a call from the delivery nurse saying we were on duty and Scott and I went to the delivery room and took turns either delivering babies or giving ether-oxygen anesthesia, using an anesthesia machine, something that we had never done before. In the second year, we had done open-drop ether anesthesia when we learned dog surgery. Unfortunately for these women, during the early stages of anesthesia they often vomited and some aspirated, occasionally causing "ether pneumonia." After the babies were delivered, they were taken to the nursery where it was our job to examine them and treat any problems they might have. Some of them became dehydrated because they would not take formula. Neither Scott nor I were able to place intravenous needles in their tiny veins, so we gave subcutaneous saline (clysis) rather than intravenous fluids. The children survived somehow. During those two weeks, working almost day and night, Scott delivered twenty-nine babies and I delivered twenty-one. We got to scrub in on cesarean sections and help with breech deliveries. It was an incredible experience. I delivered a baby boy whose mother tested positive for syphilis, as did the newborn. Both were treated with penicillin. The mother was so happy to have a son and not knowing that the child had syphilis she asked me what my name was. When I said Philip, she said "That's a wonderful name. I'm going to name this baby Philip because you delivered him."

The residents worked even harder than we did and they delivered most of the patients of the private practitioners. One obstetrician was famous for having recorded eight hundred deliveries under his name one year. He showed up late from the golf course and walked in to the delivery room in golf clothes after I had delivered the baby, held a mask over his face and said to the mother, "We brought you a beautiful baby boy, mother," and she said, "Oh, thank you doctor, you are so wonderful." However those two weeks were for both of us a huge leap in our self-confidence. What a change from the first two years of medical school!

In the fall we began our first clinical year, but not as a member of the ward team. A group of four students were assigned to a tutor whose job it was to find patients in the hospital whom we could examine. We did a complete history and physical examination, wrote up the results and presented them to the tutor, who would give us feedback to improve our performance. Our team again was Geoff Coley, Frederik Hansen, John Whitcomb and I. We were assigned, to our great fortune, to the Boston City Hospital at the Thorndike Laboratories. Our principal tutor was George Gabuzda, a young man building his reputation in liver disease. He taught us reliable history taking and physical diagnosis and was amazingly patient and thoughtful. He also took the time to search this huge hospital for the most interesting patients and took us on tours to see them. I remember seeing a patient from Cape Cod who came in with typhoid fever (due to *Salmonella typhosa*), a sailor who came in with leprosy, a 12-year-old Chinese boy who came in with liver fluke disease (due to *Clonorchis sinensis*) and many more remarkable cases. Once a week, we made rounds on patients with William Castle, the chief of the service. He was famous for isolating from the stomach a substance called "intrinsic factor" which bound vitamin B12 and made it possible for B12 to be absorbed. He was tall and imposing, with large hands which were gentle with patients. For me and many others he was inspiring as a model clinician. The other physician at the "City" whom I admired was Charles Davidson, a liver expert. He took the time to get to know lowly third-year students and became a man I could call my friend as long as he lived.

The next rotation was surgery at the Peter Bent Brigham Hospital. John Whitcomb and I were partners this time. The chief of surgery at the Brigham was Francis Daniels Moore, who was at this time in the early stage of a phenomenal career in research and in clinical surgery. He was a great favorite among the students because he gave amazing lectures, came up with memorable aphorisms and had a knack for making surgery interesting and stimulating. During the first year he gave us a clinic during which he presented a woman who had just undergone removal of her gallbladder. She was the wife of a physician but when she developed abdominal pain she had a difficult time getting her husband's serious attention. Finally she convinced him to take her to the emergency ward and the diagnosis of acute gallbladder colic or possibly acute cholecystitis was made by the surgical resident. It turned out that Dr. Moore was the husband!

We would each pick a topic in surgery and present our research paper to him and he would critique it. I chose the topic of referred pain, a major diagnostic problem, but one he had heard many times. What I learned from doing that paper helped me for the rest of my life in medicine.

We knew that research was going on in the Brigham Surgical Laboratories trying to develop a method for successfully transplanting a human kidney from one person to another while avoiding immune rejection. Unfortunately, I never got a chance to hear about this research from Dr. Joseph Murray, a plastic surgeon who led this project. Dr. Murray shared the Nobel Prize in Medicine for his success in kidney transplantation along with E. Donnall Thomas, my former hematology lab associate, for successful bone marrow transplantation. The other Brigham surgeons who taught me so well and later became my colleagues and friends were Chilton Crane in vascular surgery, John Brooks and Thomas Botsford in general surgery and Bart Quigley and Henry Banks in orthopedic surgery. In spite of the friendly atmosphere and fine teachers at the Brigham in surgery I still did not decide to become a surgeon.

During the third year, I do not recall having a course in neurology in which we met with a tutor and examined patients. This was also true of pediatrics. We had lectures and demonstrations but we needed special help with histories and physical examinations in these areas. It was not until the fourth year that we began to deal with neurology and pediatric patients. There was much wasted time in the third year. We had too many lectures, although some of the clinical lecturers were famous and great speakers. One that made a lasting impression on us was Dr. Fuller Albright, a famous endocrinologist from the Massachusetts General Hospital. He talked about his favorite topic of parathyroid diseases, but at the time we knew him, he had advanced Parkinson's disease. He had a mask-like facies and a strange high-pitched voice. When he held the long wooden pointer up to the screen where his slides were projected, his tremor would take over and the pointer would begin to go tap, tap, tap on the screen until he finally removed it. It was agonizing to see this brave man try to lecture. He later underwent experimental brain surgery, which tragically caused a severe stroke that totally impaired him for the rest of his life.

The cardiology group at the Beth Israel hospital included some of the best teachers we had. I remember particularly the lecture by Dr. Herman Blumgart in which he exercised a patient until he developed angina pectoris, ischemic heart pain, and we all saw the look of distress on the man's face before Dr. Blumgart relieved the pain with a nitroglycerin tablet. We had no patient care responsibilities until the fourth year when we found that one year was too short a time to learn so much. Years later patient care responsibilities were shifted to the third year as well and the medical students became clinical clerks on the wards.

We also had to write a paper on public health. Dave Gray, Geoff Coley, Rik Hansen and I decided that we would combine it with a trout fishing trip to Northern Vermont. Dave Gray and I wrote our paper on silicosis and complicating tuberculosis, which was occurring in the granite quarry workers near Barre, Vermont. This was my first insight into occupational diseases. We also spent time observing the practice of a family doctor in a small town in Vermont, a man who working alone did surgery, obstetrics, medicine and pediatrics, assisted only by a nurse who gave anesthesia and by a secretary. I was astounded that a man trained only in medical school and a two-year rotating internship could find the courage and skill to do so much so well.

During that third year in order to supplement my income and help pay for the costs of medical school, which were rising rapidly, I worked as a cashier every noon at the Peter Bent Brigham Hospital in the cafeteria. This gave me a meal and some cash, a chance to get to know many in the hospital and a chance for them to get to know me. I also worked in the evenings at the Department of Nutrition in the School of Public Health doing boring analyses of CO_2 and oxygen with the old Warburg apparatus. I volunteered for an experiment where I drank a pint of fat emulsion every day as a weight-gain supplement and it worked. I gained from 145 to 160 pounds in three weeks and held the weight for years.

On June 21, 1952, Marjorie Alice Lagemann and I were married in the Appleton Chapel of Harvard Memorial Church in front of all of our family and friends. Dean Sperry, who was the Pastor to the University, was suppose to marry us but he had a heart attack and at the last minute I convinced the pastor from the First Congregational Church to come over and stand in. While we were waiting to go to the altar with my best man, Eugene Dye, who was now a student at Northwestern Medical School, I began to feel lightheaded. The night before at my bachelor party I drank too much and got into a wrestling match with Scott Earle, who was a powerful man and a former ski trooper. He wrapped his legs around my chest in a scissors grip and asked me to give up. When I said no, he squeezed and broke a rib or separated the cartilages. I went to the Brigham emergency ward the next morning and they asked Dr. Bart Quigley, the orthopedic surgeon, to come and see me. He remembered me from taking care of orthopedic injuries I had in college. He laughed when he heard the story of what had happened to me. He put a large Ace bandage around my chest to splint the broken ribs but this also restricted my breathing and impaired my venous return. As it was I had a lifelong problem with fainting under stress. When we stood at the altar that afternoon, I turned gray. The minister asked us to get down on our knees and pray and in spite of this, I passed out. My bride and best man, Eugene Dye, lifted me to my feet to finish the ceremony, but I never did put the ring on Woody's finger or say "I do" when asked. My friends Rik Hansen, John Whitcomb, Dave Gray and Richmond Holder were the groom's attendants and Dorothy Whitcomb was the Matron of Honor. They have never let me forget this fiasco. As soon as Woody and Gene helped me walk down the aisle to leave, I came to, and by the time we got to the medical school for the reception in the Deanery, I was full of pep. It was a great wedding and reception except for my performance. Woody and I drove off in our newly painted black 1940 Ford sedan, which she had purchased for us. We had our honeymoon at Lake George in the cottage of a friend of hers.

My fourth year began when we returned, on July 1st, and I began neurology at Boston City Hospital. The attending physician that month was Dr. Derek Denny-Brown, a famous, awe-inspiring but kindly man who later became a good friend. The first-year resident on the team was Dr. Richard Tyler, who had been an intern at the Brigham the year before and subsequently became the chief of neurology at that hospital. I worked up great neurological cases, learning to do diagnostic procedures like visual fields and testing the bladder for denervation. I learned somewhat to read electroencephalograms (EEGs), a skill that helped me in the future. One patient I remember sadly was a man who had myasthenia gravis due to a malignant thymoma. "Louis" went in and out of total paralysis and we often had to maintain him on a respirator, the old iron lung machine. We also worked with the neurosurgeons who dealt with all kinds of emergencies coming in to the City Hospital. I read many of Dr. Denny-Brown's papers and one turned out to be fortuitous for me. He had just published on a syndrome of basilar artery aneurysm with thrombosis of the small perforating branches, which occurred in long-term hypertensive atherosclerotic patients. As a result of this month, I seriously considered making neurology my career.

The next month I took a two-month medicine rotation on the wards of Massachusetts General Hospital (MGH) on the old Bulfinch pavilion, which was a large open ward built at the turn of the 19th century. Above it was the famous Ether Dome where ether anesthesia was first used in surgery. One of the first patients that I worked up was a man with a stroke and by the time I got to him the intern and resident had both seen him and diagnosed a middle cerebral artery thrombosis. When I examined him, I found that he had neurological defects on both sides of the body in the distribution of the basilar artery and its branches. The man's picture was similar to Denny-Brown's cases which I had read about the month before. I wrote down that this old hypertensive man must have a basilar artery aneurysm with thromboses of its perforating branches, but the residents ignored my diagnosis. The man died, underwent an autopsy and the case was presented the next month as a CPC (Clinical Pathological Conference) at the MGH. These cases are published in the *New England Journal of Medicine.* The pathologist pointed out that the only person to make the correct diagnosis before death was a fourth-year medical student. By chance I had read the Denny-Brown article. More importantly I was able to trust my neurological exam and apply what I had read.

Later, I worked up a patient from a farm in Vermont who had brucellosis, caused by drinking unpasteurized milk infected by *Brucella abortis.* Shortly after taking care of him, I became ill with fever, chills and severe lower-back aches. I went to the Brigham emergency ward to see a urologist because I thought I was passing a kidney stone. Dr. Hawthorn Brown, a young urologist, examined me and said "You don't have a kidney stone. Tell me where you have been working." When he heard about my patient with brucellosis, he checked the textbook description which fit my symptoms and said, "I am going to astound those people on the medical service. I, a mere urologist, am going to admit a patient with a diagnosis of acute brucellosis." On old F-Main, the male ward, I was put in isolation and had a total workup by the intern, the resident, the chief resident, the chief of infectious disease and the chief of medicine, Dr. George W. Thorn, and no diagnosis could be arrived at. It was the second month of internship and the new interns were clumsy at doing venipunctures, putting in intravenous feedings and doing lumbar punctures. All these procedures were done on me over and over. After recovering spontaneously a week later, I found out that my discharge diagnosis was a "viral infection of unknown type," or summer disease, the same diagnosis I was given at Wisconsin General Hospital at age 16. Because of the missed time, I ended up with a poor grade in medicine at MGH.

During that summer I had obtained a job in the Massachusetts General Blood Bank working all night every fourth night cross-matching blood, releasing matched blood and drawing blood when they needed fresh whole blood. It could be very hectic at times, especially when we had to do complex cross-matches in some of the patients. One of my worst episodes occurred when fresh blood was needed and they brought in a pathology resident to donate. In those days, we drew the blood into glass bottles. I stuck the big 14 needle in his arm vein, put the bottle on the floor, removed the tourniquet and no blood flowed into the bottle. I could not understand what was wrong. He kept pumping his fist to try to get the blood to go in. Finally, I picked up the bottle to look at it and there was a huge rush of air from the bottle into his vein. It appeared that there had been an obstruction in the tubing and the air in the bottle was under pressure. It shot into his vein up into his heart where he could have died of air embolism. I remember him and me both saying, "I know you should lie on your side so that the air won't collect in your right ventricle and block the blood flow," but neither of us could remember which side to lie on. We had him turn left side down and right side up, which turned out to be correct. Nothing untoward happened other than frightening both of us until we broke out into cold sweats.

This blood bank job was a big responsibility and occasionally serious mistakes occurred. One of my three medical student coworkers was asked for a pint of blood that had already been cross-matched. He checked it out to the nurse who was going to administer the transfusion. Unfortunately, he had picked out the wrong pint of blood and the nurses also missed this error. There was a serious mismatch between the blood and the patient. Antibodies in the administered blood began to hemolyse the patient's red cells. The patient had to undergo exchange transfusions to wash out the antibodies and the hemoglobin, and luckily he did not go into renal failure. For $20 a night we often wondered whether the money was worth the risks, the stress and the sleepless nights.

During August of my fourth year we found that my wife was pregnant. Before our marriage, I had sent her for contraceptive advice to an obstetrician at the Boston Lying-In Hospital who gave us our third-year obstetrics lectures. He ended up taking care of the wives of most of the medical students. He told us before we went on our honeymoon that we should try a new contraceptive foam, which he said would be convenient and work just as well as a diaphragm. We learned later that he was testing it for a drug company. To our dismay we became pregnant and so did a number of our other classmates. We were very angry about this because we had no intention of starting a pregnancy until I had finished medical school. While I was in the Brigham hospital with the mysterious viral illness she was in the Boston Lying-In Hospital with early pregnancy bleeding and finally had a miscarriage due to what was called a "blighted ovum," a pregnancy in which the fetus never developed.

We were in poor financial shape. My job at the blood bank paid $100 a month and her salary from Perkins School for the Blind paid $175 a month. We were living in a $75 a month furnished top floor apartment near the Peter Bent Brigham Hospital at 16 Worthington Street. When we ran low on funds I would give a pint of blood for $25. During the third and the fourth year I, like many of my classmates, volunteered for research experiments to earn money and to advance scientific knowledge. There was no system in those days for informed consent. Medical students were the favorite guinea pigs of the faculty. One of the experiments I took part in was to be injected with radioactive potassium so they could follow its distribution in my body fluids with a Geiger counter and from blood and urine samples. I also was injected with my own chromium-51 labeled red cells to measure red cell volume, a pioneering and successful new method. I volunteered to receive blood that had been stored in the blood bank for three weeks to see how long the red cells would survive. This helped establish how long blood could usefully be stored in blood banks. I was always told by the faculty researchers that there were no risks. The worst experiment I ever took part in was at Massachusetts General on their research ward. They gave me a dose of vasopressin and then asked me to drink a liter of water. Vasopressin blocks the ability of the body to excrete excess water and as a result my blood pressure went up and I developed a severe headache, nausea and vomiting due to water intoxication. There was little supervision by Harvard Medical School of experiments carried out by faculty on medical students. In retrospect I see that this system was inappropriate and possibly dangerous. A medical student at the University of Washington in Seattle died of bacterial sepsis when he received a pint of old blood for red cell survival studies. It was contaminated by a cold-growing *Pseudomonas* bacterium. After this disaster the use of medical students stopped in the U.S. Now we have institutional review boards, which review every protocol for experiments done on human subjects and attempts are made to obtain truly informed consent.

We had a wonderful landlady, Mrs. O'Regan, at 16 Worthington Street in Roxbury Crossing, who lived on the first floor with her daughter. She had been born in this row house among Irish middle-class homes in the shadow of the Mission Catholic church. We lived on the third floor, which was hot in summer and cold in winter. In the fall of 1952 Woody commuted to Perkins School for the Blind in the 1940 Ford which she had purchased as a wedding present for us to replace my 1929 Model A Ford. I luckily was able to walk to most of my classes or catch a ride with other medical students who had a car. We doctors in training were what one of my friends called "the genteel poor." There were many wonderful friends who lived in our neighborhood and we helped one another whenever problems came up. John and Dottie Whitcomb, Woody's 1950 Oberlin classmates, lived on the top floor at 18 Wigglesworth Street, the next street over. Jack Hotchkiss, a classmate, and his family lived on the first floor. Phil (Oberlin 1950) and Eunice Corfman (Oberlin 1950), and Granville and Maude Coggs, the only black couple in our class, also lived on Wigglesworth. Other medical students and their wives lived nearby. Eunice and Maude took turns nursing each others' babies so they could go to work and go to classes. We got together on Friday or Saturday nights, usually in the Whitcombs' apartment, to play charades and drink Old India Ale, 25 cents a quart, the cheapest alcoholic beverage we could find.

In October and November I served a rotation in psychiatry in what was then called the Boston Psychopathic Hospital, later known as Massachusetts Mental Health Hospital. My tutor was Dr. Merrill Moore, a famous man in Boston, not only as a psychiatrist but as a published poet. When he was a student at Vanderbilt he had been part of the "Nashville Group" of American poets. When I met him, he had just published a popular book called *Clinical Sonnets.* In fact he had written and published more than 5000 sonnets, often about people he imagined from patient's stories. Someone said that he thought in sonnet form. He was a teacher with great insight. He taught the four of us in the group more than we realized. We were given one inpatient person to follow and one outpatient. We essentially did talking psychotherapy and then reported back to our tutor what had gone on in the conversation. I had an inpatient who was admitted from Harvard College with acute catatonic schizophrenia. He was a poetry student of Archibald MacLeish and was one of the most gifted undergraduates in his class. He went into a state where he was frozen in position and did not talk. My job was to go in for one hour three times a week and talk to him. Of course he never responded except with an occasional blink or grimace. I felt that I was wasting my time and his and learning nothing about him so on my own I arranged to visit his mother, who lived in a nearby town, to talk to her about her son. This turned out to be a major error on my part. She blamed herself for his schizophrenia because one of the current theories was that cold, withdrawn mothers caused the disease in their sons. However, I had also read that schizophrenia might be an hereditary disease of brain chemistry. She lodged a complaint against me and told the doctors at the psychiatric hospital that I had come to visit her. After a month of no response to any therapy they began to treat this young man with recurrent comas induced by insulin. The blood sugar would be dropped to the point of his having seizures and then he would be awakened with glucose because of some theory that this changed brain chemistry. In his case it failed to help. About the time I finished the rotation he was sent to a chronic mental disease hospital, Boston State Hospital, and became a back-ward resident. To my knowledge he never recovered from his schizophrenia. This was a total loss of a brilliant and outstanding young man. I have hated that disease ever since and wished that someone would find effective therapy for it or find some way to prevent it. Merrill Moore told me that a Nobel Prize awaited the ones who found the cause or cure for schizophrenia. That promise is still unfulfilled in 2007!

My outpatient was not a serious problem. She was the wife of a graduate student who was also in therapy because "he could not write his thesis." He had writer's block. She described what in those were days were considered classical Freudian hysterical symptoms, mostly involving sexual fantasies about her father. My outpatient instructor thought that she was a boring case and too stereotypical. I do not think that I helped her with her problem by talking with her. Now I wonder if in fact she had been sexually abused by her father and that was the cause of her frigidity with her husband. One of our group of four students had an outpatient who was a gay man, a Harvard College graduate. His chief complaint was "save my marriage." He was partnered with an aggressive, predatory homosexual man. Our patient was a faithful, passive type. The description of their life style was an eye-opener to all of us. His student therapist, who had been raised a Catholic and was extremely proper, had a difficult time relating to this pitiable homosexual man.

Every week we had staff meetings with the chief of the hospital, Dr. Harry Solomon. He was an old neurologist and psychiatrist whose specialty was the neurological complications of syphilis. I do not think he was very tuned into Freudian ideas. He always smoked cigars, listened carefully and then came out with wise and helpful suggestions on all of the patients who were presented to him. He invited our student group to his home for a picnic, with beer and great food. This was only time that I ever was a guest in the home of a Harvard Medical School faculty member. The staff at the Boston Psychopathic was wonderful. They did their best with little effective treatment other than electric shock therapy for depression. They felt almost hopeless to deal with severe psychoses like manic-depressive psychosis and schizophrenia. Psychotherapy had little effect on these severe diseases. My good friend Dr. Richmond Holder had trained at this hospital in psychiatry and he loved the place. We played squash together at Vanderbilt Hall before and after I entered medical school. I had lived for a while at 2 Otis Place close to the Charles River with him and other doctors in a wonderful top floor apartment. When I came back after the summer when I became engaged to Woody, I described the problems I had getting my family to accept her when they hoped I would marry the daughter of a rich Bostonian. After he got to know Woody he said to me one time, "Woody can only make you happy." This is one of the reasons I chose him as one of my groomsmen at my wedding.

Richmond had a house on Cape Cod at Nauset Beach. He would invite Woody and me, the Whitcombs and other friends down for weekends in the fall, winter and spring. These were wonderful breaks in our hectic lives.

In December, I served a month on the research ward called Ward 4 at Massachusetts General Hospital. I got a chance to work with many clinical investigators and help them with their experiments. This is the place where I took part in the terrible vasopressin experiment. When I worked on Ward 4 I met the student dietitian who was preparing the complicated food menus for these patients. Her name was Bobbie Pettit. I was so taken with her as an intelligent and attractive person that I told my roommate Rik Hansen about her and he began to date her. Needless to say I was so happy when they were married after medical school graduation and have had a wonderful life together. Sometimes it is fun to be a matchmaker.

I found that clinical research as it was carried out on this ward was very difficult. In those days controlled clinical trials were not popular. These were mostly intensive studies on individuals with rare diseases. I made one good friend among the research doctors, Dr. Evan Caulkins, who was a rheumatologist. It turned out that during that month I had to appear for my internship interview at Massachusetts General Hospital and he was one of the interviewers. I came into the room where there were sixteen doctors from the different specialties of the Department of Medicine sitting around a huge table. I sat next to the chief of medicine, Dr. Walter Bauer, also a rheumatologist. Dr. Bauer asked me what I thought the actions of parathyroid hormone were. I gave the standard answers according to the research by Fuller Albright, his beloved mentor at Massachusetts General. I also mentioned that parathyroid hormone had a direct effect on bone to mobilize the calcium. He asked me where I got this idea. I told him that I read it in an article by some Danish investigators. He said, "What if I tell you that we at the MGH do not believe that is true?" I replied that it was my responsibility to read the medical journals, come to my best judgment and not to take things on authority unless I knew the evidence. My friend Evan Caulkins, sitting at the far end of the table, was shaking his head at me as if to warn me not to get into any more conflicting discussions. Then the other physicians began to attack me for being such an upstart. This interview almost guaranteed that I would not get an internship at Massachusetts General. However, I still put them first on my list for a medical internship.

In January I signed up for a month on the Emergency Ward at Mass. General Hospital in the Department of Surgery. All of the patients that entered were seen first by surgeons and then triaged to medical residents if they had a medical problem. We had an interesting relationship with the local doctors in the North End of Boston. One man used to send patients after writing down a likely diagnosis on a prescription pad. He knew that the patients would be evaluated more promptly and seriously if he put down an eye-catching diagnosis. One of his favorites was to say that the patient had acute systemic lupus erythematosus, a rare disease. After a few of these referrals we caught on to his tricks. I remember an auto accident in which one of the men had been knocked unconscious, then reawakened and said that he needed to make a phone call to his family. He went to the phone booth in the emergency ward. The next minute he collapsed down on the floor of the phone booth. We ran and pulled him out. It turned out that he was again unconscious and his pupils were dilated. A rapid workup indicated that he had a skull fracture that had cut across the middle meningeal artery which runs inside the temporal bone. This artery bled between the skull and the dura, the covering of the brain (an epidural hemorrhage), causing a mass which pressed on the brain and usually caused death rapidly. He went immediately to emergency neurosurgery and survived. While I was working at the emergency ward I was still on duty every fourth night in the blood bank. I remember getting very little sleep.

We finally had to put in our priorities for internship and I listed Mass. General first, Johns Hopkins Hospital second, Barnes Hospital in St. Louis third, Peter Bent Brigham fourth and the new hospital at the University of Washington in Seattle fifth. We also found time to go for interviews. I went to the Peter Bent Brigham, where the system was to go from office to office and see about seven doctors one on one. For me this system worked nicely. I got along well with everybody, particularly the chief of medicine, Dr. George W. Thorn. One weekend my wife and I took our old 1940 Ford and drove from Boston to Baltimore in the coldest weather of the winter. We spent Friday night in a hotel and the next morning I went for an interview with the chief of medicine, Dr. A. McGee Harvey. Dr. Harvey was scheduled to give a clinical pathological conference later that morning and he seemed to be in a bad mood. As soon he heard that I was from Harvard he began to lambaste me and Harvard students in general because some were not pleased to work 24 hours a day, 365 days a year as all interns did at Johns Hopkins. I sat and listened to his tirade for half an hour and then he said that will be all. I never got a chance to say a word or answer any questions. I drove back to Boston very depressed that I had put down Johns Hopkins as my second choice for internship.

In February I had a much more relaxing month taking radiology at the Deaconess Hospital, one of the affiliated Harvard hospitals. The people who taught me were friendly and helpful. The best memory I have is attending their multi-disciplinary cancer clinic in which the patients were seen by surgeons, radiologists and oncologists. Afterwards we would sit in a group and discuss the optimal treatment for each patient. This was the best approach to team care that I had seen in medical school. In March I had a pediatric rotation at Massachusetts General. The chief resident met us the first day and took us to the laboratory, where we did blood work and urinalysis and other simple procedures, and said this is where you are going to work. The rest of that month he used us primarily for what we called "scut" work. I worked up very few patients and had a most unpleasant experience, as did my partners who were on the same rotation with me.

In April and May I took my surgical rotation at Massachusetts General Hospital. At that time I was writing, acting and rehearsing the fourth-year class show put on by the Aesculapian Club. I tended to leave early, which irritated the surgical chief resident. This rotation was a great experience particularly working in the burn unit, an area in which Massachusetts General specialized ever since the Cocoanut Grove nightclub fire of 1943. I got to scrub in at operations and hold retractors or just watch some of the most famous surgeons in the country. Finally I asked and was allowed to spend two weeks with one of the senior surgeons, Dr. Leland McKittrick, the father of my Harvard classmate Jim McKittrick. He was what we called a peripatetic surgeon, traveling from hospital to hospital seeing patients who were diagnostic problems or helping the local surgeons operate on difficult cases. As a result I got a chance to work with one of the best diagnostic and technical surgeons in Boston and one of the kindest men on the faculty.

In early April the word came out on our internships. We went to the main building at the medical school and were handed an envelope which we opened and found the good or bad news. I was not accepted by Mass General, Johns Hopkins or Barnes, where I had never taken an interview. I was accepted by the Brigham, my fourth choice. I had put the Brigham in fourth place because I was so familiar with it and it seemed so small. Later on I found out that I had struck good fortune by being accepted at the Brigham. We had a great celebration downtown in Boston at a restaurant and then got back to finishing the last few weeks of medical school.

The Aesculapian Club was 75 years old at that time. A core of fourth-year students were chosen by the students from the previous fourth year. They then elected enough classmates to total at least twenty. The purpose of this club was to put on a musical show in which the students "took off" the faculty and the medical school. I was chosen almost last among the twenty and have always suspected that it became apparent that they needed someone who could write and direct the show. I wrote new words to familiar tunes for 15 of the 20 songs in the show. I also ended up playing the female lead because no one else in the club felt comfortable playing the part of a woman. The story we concocted was rather silly. I was Lascivia, the daughter of the Ortho Contraceptive Company owner, who was a graduate of our mythical medical school that we called Missitucky Medical School, actually Harvard. Lascivia had an undiagnosed mass in her chest. She came to Missitucky Medical Center to see all of the famous doctors. After all of them failed to solve her problem, the diagnosis was made by a fourth-year medical student played by my friend David Gray. He knew what was wrong with her because he had impregnated her by oral sex nine months before. The mass in her chest was an intrathoracic pregnancy, which is of course impossible. The climax was the oral delivery of the baby! The words of the songs were raunchy and the professors at Harvard were made fools of, using our knowledge of their foibles. The cast was made up of classmates who unfortunately had little talent, including me. We did have a great piano player, however, who helped us in the rehearsals, which consisted mostly of drinking beer and smoking cigars. Finally at the beginning of June we were ready to present our great show. At the dress rehearsal my sister, Suzanne, who was then a freshman at Wellesley College, came to see the show. She was shocked by the crude medical humor that we all thought was so amusing. She had never seen her brother dressed up like a girl, singing and dancing. The second performance we gave for the class and they accepted it quite well. The third performance was performed as usual at the Longwood Cricket Club in Brookline for the faculty. We were afraid that some of our rather mean "take-offs" of faculty members would get us into trouble. I learned later that the greatest compliment we could pay a Harvard faculty member was to be mentioned in the Aesculapian show. Not to be included ever was the greater insult.

In the first week of June we graduated from medical school. It was as always a wonderful event but also sad because we were saying goodbye to classmates who were going all over the country for their internships. We knew we would not see them for a long time. My father and mother did not come to this graduation as they did not come to my Harvard College graduation. They said that they just had too many social obligations at the Country Club back in Madison. This was extremely upsetting to me. I commiserated with my friend Geoff Coley, whose parents did not come for the same superficial reasons.

After graduation Woody and I drove the old car to Indianapolis to visit her family, then to Madison to visit my family. We then drove to northern Wisconsin for a second honeymoon. We visited the now-empty Snodgrass family cottage on a lake and stayed in my Uncle Tom's cabin on a trout stream. I returned just before July 1 to find that all of the other interns at the Brigham had been told to begin a week before. One of the previous interns had to stay on my ward and cover for me during that week. He and Don Thomas, the outgoing chief resident, were justifiably furious with me and I got off to a bad start of my internship in medicine at the Brigham.

3

Internship

✦

1953–1954

When I arrived at the Peter Bent Brigham Hospital for my internship I found myself one of ten new medical interns, all that the Department of Medicine selected in 1953. Among my fellow interns were the following people from my Harvard Medical School class: John G. Harter, Stanley James Adelstein, Philip Bromberg, Buris R. Boshell, and Barbara M. Orski, the latter being one of the first female interns taken at the Brigham in medicine. The other interns were George F. Cahill Jr., who came from Columbia Medical School, Arnold Golodetz from Rochester School of Medicine, Frederick Luft from the University of Washington School of Medicine and Frank I. Marcus from Boston University. Fred Luft was a member of the first graduating class from the new medical school at the University of Washington in Seattle.

The schedule of work was traditional at most academic teaching hospitals throughout the country. It was called "every other night and weekend." For example, I would come in on Saturday morning, work all day, all night, all day Sunday, Sunday night and Monday until 5:00 or 6:00 in the evening and then have the evening off at home where I usually fell asleep over supper. Tuesday morning I would arrive on the ward at 6:30 a.m., work 24 hours and get off Wednesday evening. Thursday was the same, work all night and get off Friday evening. Saturday and Sunday I would be free to recover before the next week's schedule. Our support system consisted of a senior assistant resident working with two interns on one ward during the day. Our senior residents were Donald M. Haskins, Albert E. Renold, Eugene D. Robin and Leonard S. Sommer. Every other night the senior resident covered our ward and admitted new patients from the emergency ward. One of the six junior assistant residents admitted patients on alternate nights and a senior resident from another ward covered us for the old patients. I have calculated that the number of hours worked per week averaged one hundred and thirty-two by this system! At the present time because of scandals which occurred in New York city where interns and residents made serious errors allegedly due to lack of sleep, it is mandated throughout the United States that interns and residents work no more than every third night and third weekend and average no more than eighty hours on duty a week.

We were paid a salary of twenty-five dollars a month for the privilege of working this hard. Twenty years before 1953 all the interns lived at the hospital, were single, and received room, board and laundry; the twenty-five dollars was supposed to be enough for incidentals. By 1953 the majority of interns were married and the wives had to support them while they went through this program. Thus the training program at the Peter Bent Brigham Hospital was being subsidized by the work of the wives of these trainees. This system put tremendous stress on those of us who went through it. I clearly remember being awakened in the middle of the night by a telephone call from one of the wards and a nurse telling me of a problem. I prescribed some medication over the phone and fell asleep again. The next morning when I came to the ward the head nurse asked me to co-sign the order in the prescription order book but I did not remember giving that order. Fortunately such middle of the night, wake-up decisions turned out to be correct most of the time.

Partly as a punishment for being late for my internship, I was assigned to F-Main, the main male public ward, which usually contained thirty beds. One senior resident and two interns cared for this large number of patients. At night we had a third-year nursing student from the Brigham School of Nursing caring for the patients and we had a rotating staff nurse available on call if she and I got into trouble. It was an incredible workload for the nurses to take care of this many patients. The distribution of beds on the ward as we walked in from the hall was as follows: there were double rooms on the right and on the left side, then two single rooms, which we used as our "intensive care rooms," then a small ward containing eight patients who were moderately ill and a sixteen-bed circular ward where the patients were supposed to be less ill. There were no intensive care or cardiac care units on the medical services in 1953. The workday began at 6:00 or 6:30 in the morning with what we called work rounds, where the senior resident and the two interns, the head nurse, and often a staff nurse saw every patient and reviewed the results from the previous day. The interns wrote notes in the charts of their patients and most importantly wrote orders for that day. We only had a few minutes to talk with each patient, do a quick and focused physical examination, discuss his situation (at the end of the patient's bed) and then make decisions on what to do for him that day. The senior resident left at 8:00 a.m. to meet with the chief of the medical service, Dr. George W. Thorn or whoever was substituting for him, between 8:00 and 8:30 in an exercise called morning report. The resident would tell Dr. Thorn briefly who was admitted, what their problems were and what they were going to do about them. The resident described any deaths, untoward accidents or anything else that the chief should know. The interns meanwhile were examining patients, writing orders and filling out forms to order tests.

At 8:30 we all went to the X-ray department to review the films of our patients that had been taken during the previous day. The staff attending physician assigned to our ward that month often met with us in the X-ray department. These "attendings" were full-time academic doctors attached to the staff at the Peter Bent Brigham Hospital or they were doctors in private practice in the nearby city who had admitting privileges at the Brigham. Legally they were responsible for each patient. After we presented the history and physical findings of each new patient the attending was supposed to talk to the patient briefly, examine him and write an attending note in which he either agreed with our diagnoses and our care plan or amended or changed our plans. Being an attending physician on a busy ward where three to eight patients were admitted every night was a challenging job considering that the morning rounds were over at 12:00 noon when we all went to a teaching conference in the amphitheater.

The X-ray conference on noon Tuesday was a highlight of the week because Dr. Merrill Sosman served as master of ceremonies. He was a great teacher and most of the senior staff attended. On Friday morning surgical grand rounds were held from 10:00 to 11:00 a.m. and medical grand rounds immediately thereafter, between 11:00 and 12:00. Dr. Francis D. Moore, the chief of surgery, played grand inquisitor of the speakers and of the senior staff surgeons. It was compulsory for us to attend medical rounds but I always tried to attend surgical rounds, where I enjoyed the show and learned a great deal of what I know about surgical practice. Dr. Thorn played a less active role in Medical Rounds, leaving the choice of topics and speakers to the chief medical resident, and the questions to the audience.

There were also subspecialty conferences at noon other days in the week. We then all rushed off to lunch in the cafeteria. When we returned to the ward at about 1:30 p.m. we began to write discharge medications and orders to get patients out of the hospital so that the new admissions that were waiting in the emergency ward or the outpatient department could be brought in. All afternoon we did diagnostic procedures on patients such as lumbar punctures or tapping fluid from the chest or abdomen and doing workups on the new patients. Supper was at 6:00 p.m. and as brief as possible. We then went back to the wards and worked until midnight, admitting new patients who were already waiting on the ward or were being sent up from the emergency ward. We all gathered at midnight in the cafeteria for an evening snack. Here great tales were told by the residents and the private physicians who were visiting their own patients. I learned more good medical stories at midnight snacks than I ever heard in daily rounds. From 1:00 to 6:00 a.m. we were usually up admitting patients, doing procedures, and occasionally sneaking one or two hours of sleep. F-Main had a small office for members of the psychiatry department and we took to sleeping on the patient's couch because the nurses could get to us in a minute or two.

Grand rounds in medicine at the Brigham were a great occasion. The chief resident chose the cases and the topics and picked the speakers, which was an incredible amount of responsibility to give to a person who was just finishing his training. The chief resident could invite anyone in Boston to come and speak at our medical grand rounds. It was considered an honor to be asked. X-ray conference at the Brigham was outstanding because Dr. Merrill Sosman was the chief of radiology and one of the greatest diagnostic radiologists in Boston history. He used to play games with the audience, asking the senior doctors and senior residents what they thought the X-rays showed. After all had committed themselves, then he would show us what we missed and make us look mildly foolish. The surgical grand rounds were exciting because Dr. Frances D. Moore, the chairman of the department, insisted that all of his division chiefs be there. A lively discussion was encouraged and he would challenge the senior surgeons' opinions. The only surgeon bright and confident enough to challenge Dr. Moore was Dr. J. Engelbert Dunphy, who unfortunately left in 1954 to be chief of surgery at the Harvard service of Boston City Hospital. Later he became the chairman of surgery at the University of California Medical School at San Francisco. He and Dr. Moore were both knowledgeable and witty. It was a performance I would have paid to watch.

On my first night alone on F-Main two patients died and I had a number of admissions. One was a young man with diabetic ketoacidosis and coma, which I had never treated alone before. If it had not been for Dr. Warren E. C. Wacker, an assistant resident from George Washington University, helping me I could not have made it through that first night. At the first of our mortality conferences, which occurred once a week, I presented all five patients who died and received rather sharp criticism from some of the senior doctors in the front row who did not know the details of the patients' problems. These "death rounds" were supposed to be helpful by correcting errors and improving the management of patients but often the criticisms were unjustified and left me angry and frustrated.

My senior resident on F-Main was Eugene Robin, a very intelligent man who was older than the rest of us. He had just finished two years doing research in the pulmonary lab at the Brigham. Dr. Robin was justifiably concerned that we perform well on F-Main but he was prone to criticize every little detail of management that he thought we had missed. John Harter, my classmate, was my co-intern. John had a great deal of self-confidence, was quite knowledgeable, fought hard for his patients' welfare and did not like to take advice. One time Dr. Robin questioned his motives about the care of a patient who had done badly. John lost his temper, picked up Gene by his tie and the collar of his shirt, lifted him up against the wall and threatened to punch him out if he ever questioned his motives again.

I however was full of the theory but weak on the practice of medicine. I needed specific instructions about which medications to give, in what doses and how often. For example there were different schedules for giving people digitalis, slowly in those in mild heart failure or rapidly for those in acute heart failure. I also was not skilled at putting in intravenous feeding lines and had to learn the tricks of this trade. After three weeks on F-Main with many deaths in patients that I was caring for and a good deal of criticism by Eugene Robin I became discouraged and depressed. I did not realize at that time that most of the patients I took care of were in the end stage of diseases like leukemia, severe coronary artery disease, renal failure and pulmonary failure and they were going to die no matter what we did for them. One time I forgot to prescribe a laxative to an old man who had suffered multiple heart attacks. While we were making morning rounds he died sitting on a bedpan, straining to have a bowel movement. Dr. Robin in frustration and anger said that I had "killed that man." I then went to my chief resident, Richard Gorlin, and told him that I had better resign as an intern because I was not good enough to satisfy the demands placed on me at the Brigham. He tried to reassure me and told me "Phil, you expect too much of yourself. Here at the Brigham we do not expect anyone to be 100 percent perfect; 95 percent perfect is good enough." I thanked him for this reassurance, went home and talked to my wife about whether or not I should quit. We both agreed that I should not resign and I went on with the internship. Later as a resident and a chief resident, I helped other interns go through similar crises of confidence. When Warren Wacker was admitting patients to F-Main he helped me to deal with practical problems and gave me the confidence to handle these sick people in the middle of the night. We became friends from this shared experience and have remained close friends to this day. By the end of the month I began to trust my physical examinations and found that I could keep up with the details of care of all of my fifteen to eighteen patients. I even made a few diagnoses that nobody else considered.

One patient I cared for will illustrate the primitive conditions of our work. We admitted an FBI agent with severe chest pain from Fenway Park, where he had been watching a Red Sox game. Although only 32 years of age, his electrocardiogram (EKG) showed the pattern of an acute myocardial infarction or "heart attack." I remember Gene Robin saying, "I cannot believe it, this man is younger than I am." We put him in the double room at the end of the ward because there was no such thing as a coronary care unit, and tried to make things quiet and restful for him. Unfortunately someone forgot to secure the strap around the tall oxygen tank next to his bed. The oxygen tank fell over and broke the top off the tank and the oxygen began to shoot out like a jet stream. This made the huge oxygen tank spin round and round, crashing into everything in the room. We found the patient standing on his bed calling for help. What a way to treat a patient with an acute heart attack! He survived in spite of this episode and returned to duty.

I am now amazed how little in those days we could do when somebody had a cardiac arrest. We would be called by the nurses, run to the room, and if we could hear no heart sounds, pound on the chest to stimulate the heart to contract. If the EKG showed no electrical activity or the rhythm disturbance known as ventricular fibrillation we would inject epinephrine directly into the heart. Rarely did we ever resuscitate anyone successfully. Cardiopulmonary resuscitation (CPR) had not been developed yet. Then our job was to pronounce the patient dead, talk to the family when they came in and make sure that we got autopsy permission if possible.

The Brigham in those days obtained autopsies on 80 percent of the patients who died. We learned a great deal from these autopsies. We found out what we had missed while the patients were still alive and we often learned the reasons why these patients died. I remember many obese patients laid open on the autopsy table with abdominal fat hanging over the edge of the table, lungs that were gray-black from smoking instead of pink, narrowing of all of the coronary arteries by cholesterol plaques and a fresh clot in one of the main heart arteries. The combination of obesity, smoking, high cholesterol and often diabetes causes this coronary atherosclerosis and kills Americans to this day.

During this month my wife, Woody, was working at a settlement house in Dorchester which earned us a bit more income. This job was an interesting teaching experience which contrasted with her teaching the blind students at Perkins. In July we found out that she was pregnant again but at 10 weeks she began to bleed heavily, was admitted to the Boston Lying-In Hospital and miscarried again. This was a male fetus that looked normal but had not developed a placenta. In the recovery period Woody developed acute narrow-angle glaucoma in both eyes because they had given her atropine when they did a dilatation and curettage after the miscarriage. She was quite nearsighted and dilating the pupil with atropine is a known risk factor for such people. I could get no one to pay attention to her eyes with their bulging, steamy corneas, which I immediately recognized as acute glaucoma. I had to ask one of the senior physicians at the Brigham, Dr. Eugene Eppinger, to call her obstetrician and insist that he get an ophthalmologist to see her. By the time we finally got the specialist to see her, the glaucoma had resolved mostly on its own. This was the second bad experience that she and I had with obstetric doctors, who seemed to have limited competence in anything outside of their narrow field of obstetrics and gynecology. Fortunately I was assigned to an early vacation at the end of August and we went back to Lake George, where we had had our honeymoon a year before, and joined two other couples for a wonderful one-week vacation. Woody continued to worry that she would be an "habitual aborter" and would never have a live baby. After we came home from vacation she returned to teach her fourth year at Perkins School for the Blind.

I moved to the semiprivate service on F-Second in September. F-Second was a sixteen-bed ward staffed by a junior resident and one intern, paired with E-Second, which was the female semiprivate ward just across the bridge. My new fellow intern was George Cahill, whom I found to be one of the brightest people I have known, very skillful at procedures and efficient. He often came to my ward about four in the afternoon and told me that everything was "shipshape" and he was going to go home early. I would check his patients with him and everything seemed to be calm. Within an hour after he left some of his patients began to develop acute problems and I would spend the night doing diagnostic and therapeutic procedures on his patients. I never did figure out how he could calm down his ward temporarily so that he could leave early. I had trouble ever getting out of the hospital by six or seven in the evening.

My ability to deal with patients was better after the months on F-Main. The staff and private physicians admitted patients to F-Second and I had to deal with each of these doctors individually as they came to see their private patients. I began to learn which doctors I could trust and which ones' patients the resident and I needed to take charge of. In October I served as intern on E-Second, the female semiprivate ward.

In November and December I moved to the main public female ward, E-Main, where my senior resident was Albert Renold and my co-intern was George Cahill. The ward was exactly the same size and arrangement as F-Main. Albert Renold was from Geneva, Switzerland. He already had some training as an endocrinologist there and he had recently worked with George Thorn in his laboratory in the Brigham. George Cahill, whose interest even then was in biochemistry, diabetes and intermediary metabolism, eventually went on to the Joslin Diabetes Clinic at the Deaconess Hospital. Working at the clinical research center at the Peter Bent Brigham in the 1960s he carried out landmark studies on the adaptation of obese human subjects to prolonged fasting. These are still considered classics in the intermediary metabolism literature. He then went on to be an administrator in the Howard Hughes Medical Research Institute and has become emeritus professor from Harvard Medical School. Albert Renold went back to Geneva, where he became chief of endocrinology at the medical school there and later president of the European Diabetes Association.

The workload on E-Main was as difficult if not more so than F-Main. The female patients were often in their 80s, had multiple organ diseases and were frail and difficult to care for. An exception to this type of patient occurred when a young woman was transferred from the Boston Lying-In Hospital after the delivery of her first child. She developed acute renal failure for reasons not clear to us and was placed on conservative renal failure management, in which the Brigham specialized. The kidney specialists did not choose to use their single, newly developed kidney dialysis machine to help this woman. She became more and more uremic and finally developed a distended abdomen full of fluid, called ascites. To give her some comfort I was asked to drain the fluid. After carefully sterilizing the skin I put in a large needle and drained off the fluid. The fluid cultured a *Pseudomonas* bacterium and within 24 hours she developed full-blown peritonitis due to this *Pseudomonas* organism, which was resistant to all antibiotics, and she died. I cared a great deal about this young woman and wanted so much to see her survive. We kept hoping that her kidneys would open up but a biopsy of one of the kidneys showed destruction of all of the urine filtering units, the glomeruli. At death rounds when I presented her case some of the faculty physicians in the front row accused me of causing the peritonitis which led to her death. Other staff doctors pointed out that the bacterium was present in the fluid already and that uremic patients were unusually prone to develop infections.

John Harter joined me on E-Main in December. He cared for a black woman who was a teacher at Boston Latin School and had had a stroke which paralyzed her right side and left her unable to talk. We fed her by a tube from her nose to her stomach. She kept pulling out the tube with her left hand and shook her head as if to say no when we replaced it. We restrained her left arm. After three weeks and no sign of recovery we sent her to a nursing home. We were told that after two days there she aspirated her tube feedings and died. We rarely considered whether patients wanted to be kept alive against their will in those days. By the New Year of 1954 I was in a state of exhaustion from these demanding rotations.

Luckily for me, in January and February I was scheduled to the emergency ward every other night and every other weekend. The emergency ward was not as rigorous as the wards. The Brigham emergency ward was small and rather primitive by modern standards. We drew patients from the surrounding Roxbury area, Jamaica Plain and Brookline. Some of the patients who were brought in by ambulance were very ill but many of the patients just walked in to get help with minor complaints like a cold or a sore throat. There was no separate walk-in clinic at night. We came to know many of the emergency ward repeaters. For example, one unfortunate man had suffered four heart attacks from severe coronary disease and had chest pain on the least exertion. His record contained about two hundred visits to the emergency ward in a year. We also had a group of asthmatics who kept coming in with repeated attacks. We put them in bed, inserted an intravenous line and began infusing them with saline. We then mixed the drugs which we used to treat the asthma in another bottle of saline and brought it to the bedside so we could hook it up to the infusion. I often found the patients already breathing easier after they had received nothing but saline. From this I concluded that there was a large emotional component to flare-ups of asthma.

I enjoyed working with the surgical residents on patients involving both of our areas of expertise. The nurses attempted to triage patients to the correct service, medicine or surgery, but often cases were confusing and I would end up seeing a patient with an acute surgical abdomen. I noticed that Boston or Brookline police tended to park outside the entrance and come in and out of the emergency ward, especially at night. I came to realize that they were there to keep order and to protect the nurses from any threatening patient. I remember one man came in drunk, cursed one of our nurses and then hit her. The policemen took him outside and two or three of them worked him over with their Billy clubs, I could hear the "thump, thump," and the "ouch, ouch" as they taught him a lesson. He came back in the emergency ward and gave us no more trouble.

We had about one month rotating through the medical clinics with more nights off, unless we had to help in the emergency ward. One of our duties was to work in the syphilis clinic, actually called Lues Clinic, an old name for syphilis. There we saw many patients with tertiary syphilis who had been treated too late and had developed aortic heart valve insufficiency, tabes dorsalis or dementia. We also saw new cases of syphilis with penile chancres and occasionally secondary syphilis with a rash on the palms and soles and over the rest of the body. We learned how to diagnose new cases of syphilis in the clinic by looking at tissue juice through a dark field microscope for the spirochetes (*Treponema palidum*). Of course we also used a serological (blood) test for syphilis.

My last rotation in late April, May, and early June was on the private service, which consisted of three wards, A-Main, A-Second and A-Third, where we took care of the patients sent in by private staff doctors. The doctor I enjoyed working with the most was Samuel A. Levine, a cardiologist. I found out later that he had been the first Harvard medical student to take a rotation at the new Peter Bent Brigham Hospital. He was a fine teacher about patient care and physical examination and a great storyteller. One of my favorite stories by Dr. Levine came from his experiences in the Army. He was drafted in World War I and sent to France just as the war ended in 1918. Shortly after arriving there the great influenza pandemic broke out and was particularly bad among the soldiers who were still remaining in Europe. Since he was the most junior person on the staff of the military hospital he had to give "hands-on" care to the patients. The doctors and nurses were not immune from influenza and they were also dying. Every morning he came in they would say, "How do you feel today Dr. Levine?" and he would say, "Fine, I feel fine." Finally they pulled him aside and the nurses said "We do not understand. You get exposed to influenza more than anybody else in this hospital and yet you never catch it. What is your secret?" Dr. Levine remarked as a joke, "I smoke Pall Mall cigarettes and the smoke seems to kill the virus." The next morning everybody in the hospital was smoking Pall Malls.

One of Dr. Levine's prior fellows was a doctor at Georgetown Medical School named Proctor Harvey. He and Dr. Levine wrote a book called *Clinical Auscultation of the Heart,* based on correlations among the physical examination, the electrocardiogram and phonocardiograms (recordings of heart sounds). It became a bible for me and my fellow interns and residents because it explained clearly what we should hear and why. Among the many outstanding cardiology fellows who came to train with him was Bernard Lown, who was there during my internship. He subsequently went on to practice with Dr. Levine and helped to found International Physicians for Prevention of Nuclear War. He and the other physicians in the group were awarded the Nobel Peace Prize. Dr. Levine taught me how to use morphine when it came time to ease the death of end-stage patients. I particularly remember a young man dying of tight aortic stenosis before cardiac surgery was possible. He was extremely short of breath, his hands and feet were turning black due of lack of cardiac output and his kidneys had shut down. Dr. Levine told me to keep giving him morphine until he did not suffer anymore and he died in peace. When I was seeing patients in my weekly medical clinic, a black lady brought in her 9-year old son with a complaint of classical angina pectoris (chest pain) on exertion. No one would believe that a child could have ischemic heart pain, so I called Dr. Levine and told him the story. He said the boy probably had an aberrant right coronary artery coming off the pulmonary artery instead of the aortic root, so his heart was getting blue blood low in oxygen and causing ischemic chest pain. No treatment was then available for this developmental error and no coronary angiograms were possible to confirm Dr. Levine's diagnosis.

Another doctor on the staff was Dr. William P. Murphy, an elderly man who sent many patients in to the private service. When he was young he had the good fortune to work with George Richards Minot at the Thorndike Laboratory at City Hospital. He helped Dr. Minot grind up liver and feed it to patients through a stomach tube to treat pernicious anemia, which Dr. Minot thought was due to a deficiency of some essential food substance which we now know is vitamin B-12. At the same time George Whipple in Rochester, New York, was working on the same project. In 1926 these three succeeded in turning pernicious anemia from a fatal disease to a treatable one. All three shared the Nobel Prize for Medicine in 1934. A crude liver extract was developed that could be injected into the muscles, and later purified vitamin B-12 by injection became the standard treatment. Dr. Murphy had developed a huge private practice. It seemed as if every patient he admitted also had pernicious anemia and was coming to him for monthly liver extract injections. He sent in an elderly woman who was in heart failure that we treated. Her record said that she had pernicious anemia and needed her monthly liver extract. One morning before breakfast I took a nasogastric tube and slipped it down her esophagus into the stomach, removed some of the stomach contents and measured its acidity. It was pH 3, a normal acidity. I sent it to the laboratory for an acid analysis, which was also normal. Pernicious anemia was usually caused by atrophy of the acid cells of the stomach that produced the protein which was necessary for B-12 absorption. Such patients had no stomach acid. I wrote a note in the chart saying that this patient seemed miraculously to have had a spontaneous remission of her pernicious anemia. When Dr.

Murphy saw what I had done he was furious and he went to Dr. Thorn and complained angrily. Dr. Thorn called me in and explained that it was the job of the interns and residents to care for Dr. Murphy's patients because he was no longer capable of managing difficult medical problems. He also pointed out that everybody knew that most of these patients did not have pernicious anemia but there was little we could do to undo their belief in his diagnosis. He told me he did not want me to embarrass Dr. Murphy again and I did what he said.

We had another elderly physician, Dr. J. P. O'Hare, an excellent internist who had been a pioneer in studying treatment of hypertension in the 1930s. He published a famous paper in the *Journal of Clinical Investigation* in which he treated malignant hypertension, a uniformly fatal disease, with intravenous nitroprusside. This potent vasodilator dropped the blood pressure to normal and for three weeks the patients did beautifully but then they began to develop side effects from the nitroprusside and it had to be stopped. In those days there was no other medication to control the blood pressure.

One of the most impressive doctors on the staff was Dr. C. Sidney Burwell. I knew him as a doctor who was an expert in heart and pulmonary problems and I later found out that he was an expert in heart and lung complications of pregnancy. I also learned that he had been dean of the medical school from 1935 to 1949 and later was named the first Samuel A. Levine Professor of Medicine. When he retired he wrote one of the definitive books on heart disease in pregnancy. He was famous for a statement that he allegedly made to the graduating class during his tenure as dean. He said, "Half of what we have taught you is wrong. Unfortunately we do not know which half is the wrong half." This story is told in the book called *Medicine at Harvard: The First 300 Years* by Drs. H. Beecher and M. Altschule. I helped care for a patient that Dr. Burwell had followed for many years, a woman with tuberculous pericarditis. Her heart was encased in calcified scar tissue from the treated tuberculosis and it was impairing the blood flow into the heart, causing her a form of low-output heart failure. She was too fragile to undergo the extensive surgery needed to remove the calcified pericardium and she died while on my service.

Another doctor who was important in my intern year was John P. Merrill, who was chief of the renal division at the Brigham. With the help of Dr. Carl Walter, a Brigham surgeon, and his engineers at Walter's Fenwall company, he improved upon a dialysis machine called an artificial kidney that was invented by Dr. Kolff in Holland. This machine could keep patients alive who had developed acute kidney failure. He also used it to support patients undergoing renal transplantation using cadaver kidneys, which Dr. Moore, Dr. David Hume and Dr.

Joseph Murray were pioneering on the surgical service. We helped care for some of these patients on the medical wards. All of the transplants of cadaver kidneys failed until some years later when better immunosuppressive drugs were developed. In 1954, however, the first successful human renal transplantation was carried out between identical twins because no immune rejection was possible in such twins. Dr. Murray shared the Nobel Prize in Medicine for his work in renal transplantation with E. Donnall Thomas for his work in bone marrow transplantation. Don Thomas had been a chief resident at the Brigham and a fellow worker with me in Dr. Clement Finch's laboratory.

Dr. George Thorn made rounds on his private patients early in the morning. We met on A-Third, presented our patients to him that we had worked up during the previous afternoon and night and then listened anxiously while he took a further history and examined the patients. Once he asked me what my examination of a man's testicles showed. I had to admit that I had neglected to examine the man's testicles. His expression was so disapproving that I never forgot to examine a man's testicles again. Dr. Thorn had many patients sent in with vague complaints of fatigue, weakness and lassitude who had been worked up thoroughly at the Mayo Clinic and other academic medical centers but were not satisfied. They were sent to the Brigham because someone thought they might have mild adrenal insufficiency, the area where Dr. Thorn was the world expert. When we finally ruled out adrenal insufficiency he would then give them a placebo consisting of one small potassium tablet every day, telling them that their potassium was a little low. Then he would send them home, quite happy with his evaluation. Dr. Thorn was always kind and rarely critical of his patients or of his young interns and residents. He had one famous problem, however, and that was difficulty remembering the names of his interns and residents, or even his medical staff physicians. When one of his young protégés was made chairman of medicine at a new medical school, Dr. Thorn allegedly said in tribute, "We will never forget old what's his name."

When late June arrived I was asked to stay on and work an extra week serving as a senior resident on the private service to make up for my late arrival at the beginning of the year. This was actually a good experience and I learned how to help new interns adjust to their first week.

During January and February I had been notified that I would likely be drafted into the armed forces. At that time there was a doctors' draft and if you did not volunteer you would be drafted, usually into the Army. The Korean War was still going on. I discussed this with Dr. Eugene Eppinger, who was the house staff advisor. He advised me to enlist in the Navy and not in the Army. I took his advice and enlisted, filled out the papers and was sworn in at the end of June as a Lieutenant Junior Grade in the United States Naval Reserve. The first thing I did was buy used blue and khaki uniforms from a friend who had already served in the Navy. As I left the Brigham on June 30, 1954, I went to Chelsea Naval Hospital on the east side of Boston for some training in surgery. I had been given orders to go on a destroyer minelayer off the coast of China for the next two years and I would have to learn how to take out an appendix because I would be the only doctor in the group of four destroyers. I went to the operating room and had scrubbed in on an appendectomy when I got a call from the commanding officer at the hospital. I came to his office and he said, "There is an emergency. Your orders have been changed. You are going immediately to Kingsville, Texas, to the Naval Auxiliary Air Station there, where they are very short of help." So I went home and told Woody the good news that I would not be leaving her for two years.

4

U.S. Navy Medical Reserve

◆

1954–1956

I flew from Boston to Corpus Christi, Texas, on July 2, 1954, and then took a bus to Kingsville, where I checked in at the Kingsville Naval Auxiliary Air Station at 6:00 p.m. The Marine officer asked me, "How long have you been in the Navy?" and I said "Twenty-four hours." He said, "I can tell. You have put your collar bars [of a lieutenant junior grade] on horizontally and they should be vertically on the collar." I laughed and said, "I have a lot to learn about the Navy." He called Commander N, the regular Navy doctor in charge of the dispensary, who said to me: "Doctor, we are exhausted here because Dr. Stanley Wiener and I have had to stand port and starboard duty for weeks and we need relief." He meant relief for himself as I found out later. He never stood duty again in the next two years I served there and was famous in the Navy for avoiding duty whenever possible. The Kingsville NAAS had only a dispensary, not a naval hospital, with a ward that contained ten beds and rarely more than one or two patients. There was a large area where sick call was held three times a day. I found out that I was on duty July 3rd and 4th, while the Commander and Dr. Wiener rested up. If it hadn't been for the experience of the senior hospital corpsmen, who had served in action in Korea, guiding me I would have never known what to do.

Stanley Wiener had been trained as a flight surgeon in Pensacola, Florida. His medical training was in internal medicine plus a year of training in cardiology in California. He was intelligent and competent, but angry at being on duty at Kingsville, Texas. He wanted out of the Navy as soon as possible. His wife, Norma, and he had recently had a first baby, a girl born with a severe cleft lip and palate who was having a difficult time feeding. They wanted to go home to Denver, where she could have surgeries to repair this. He explained that Commander

N, a flight surgeon, collected flight pay by flying around the base four hours a month, but never rode the helicopter to any of the plane crashes which occurred often. Dr. N ordered me to go out on his crash coverage turns even though I was not a flight surgeon and earned no flight pay.

On July 4th, I was on duty at night when a loud alarm went off and an ambulance pulled up in front of the dispensary. The corpsman driver said, "That alarm is for you, Doc. Jump in. We are going out to a crash site." We drove into the King Ranch, which encircles Kingsville, trying to find where a plane had crashed. We knew the general vicinity because we could look up and see planes circling around the site but the radio in our ambulance could not communicate with the radios in the planes up above us. Finally, after going down dead-end roads and cutting some fences, we reached the crash site. Unfortunately, it was mostly a hole in the ground, at the bottom of which was burning magnesium from parts of the plane. It was our job to collect body parts of the dead pilot for identification. He had been returning from a cross-country flight to California when something went wrong and he could not make it to the base or eject from the aircraft. We found his helmet and inside it was half of his brain and skull. We also found bits and pieces of his body in the bushes and a good part of his burned body and we put them all in a rubber body bag and took them back to the base to identify. We were able to get a fingerprint from a tip of one finger and part of his jaw for dental records. To my surprise and sorrow, the pilot was a young man named Burwell, the son of Langdon Burwell, a physician on Cape Cod whom I knew and the grandnephew of C. Sidney Burwell, my professor and teacher at the Brigham Hospital. The horrible smell of burned and rendered human fat and flesh was almost more than I could take and I thought I was going to faint. The corpsman told me, "Doc, you don't look too good. Go out and let us finish this unpleasant job."

Kingsville Naval Auxiliary Air Station was a satellite field of the U.S. Navy Advanced Air Training Command at Corpus Christi. The other satellite auxiliary airfield was in Beeville, Texas. Our base contained two fields. South Field was for training in propeller-driven planes, where student pilots learned instrument flying and tactics and went to ground school. They then graduated to the North Field, where they learned to fly jet aircraft, first in two-seat trainers with an instructor and then solo in Grumman F-111 fighters, which were second-line carrier aircraft at that time and used for training. Pilots did their primary training in Pensacola, Florida. After going through a year of advanced training in south Texas they went to California to qualify for landing on aircraft carriers at sea. I was shocked to learn that overall 10 percent of those who started training in

Pensacola had been killed in accidents before they qualified for carrier landings. The base was the largest airfield in the Navy and contained about ten thousand Navy personnel and their families. There was a large housing development for married officers just outside the base, where Marjorie and I would live. On the base there was housing for the married enlisted men consisting of trailer homes. Single men lived in barracks.

I alone took care of the enlisted men who came to sick call at 8 a.m., 1 p.m., and 6 p.m. I also took care of women and children, who came in at any time of day. Stan Wiener, as a flight surgeon, saw the officers. He and I alternated night coverage. Commander N saw no patients. He sat in his office and "pushed paper."

The town of Kingsville itself was about ten thousand in population. It was the headquarters of the King Ranch, which extended all the way to the Mexican border and was one of the largest ranches in the world. I found myself doing pediatrics although I had had only a one-month rotation in this specialty in medical school. I ran an obstetrics clinic with the help of two skillful registered Navy nurses, seeing fifty patients twice a week. Our job was to make sure that their pregnancies developed normally and that we got them to the Corpus Christi Naval Hospital in time for delivery. If we did not time it correctly, then it was my job to deliver them at the dispensary. I also ended up doing orthopedics and minor surgery. In both areas, I was poorly trained. The only area where I felt confident was in general internal medicine. The weather in Kingsville was very hot in the summer, 90°F by 9 a.m., and over 100°F most of the day. The only air conditioning in the dispensary was in the Commander's office. Our dispensary was a one-story building with a flat black tar roof that collected the heat. Almost every afternoon dust storms blew in from the Gulf of Mexico, making flying dangerous. In the winter the weather cooled off in hours to 40° from 80°F depending on the frequency of cold weather fronts which came in from the north. These "Northers" brought many men to sick call with asthma attacks. Kingsville was at the end of the Navy supply chain, both for medical equipment and for aircraft maintenance. On a number of occasions, we ran out of common antibiotics, wound dressings and even aspirin.

My wife, Woody, flew down to Kingsville the first week after I arrived, after closing our apartment in Boston, selling our car and packing our things in big wooden boxes. Her trip was difficult for a woman who was seven months pregnant. They did not serve food on the plane. She could not get food when they stopped to change planes. She became dehydrated and starved and began to panic because our baby quit moving in her womb. When she arrived at Corpus Christi,

Norma Wiener and I met her with Norma's car. Without stopping for lunch we drove into Corpus to buy a Plymouth station wagon, furniture for the apartment, a bed and a big air conditioner for the living room, all on credit. Norma drove Woody back to Kingsville, gave her a snack and let her take a nap. I drove back in our new car and found a place for dinner and we stayed in a motel with air conditioning. Woody and the baby somehow survived the terrible ordeal. In two days we moved into a new apartment in the Navy housing project. We were fortunate that a skilled obstetrician named Heywood Walling had moved from North Carolina to practice in Kingsville because he loved the hunting and the ranch country. Woody had only gained from 126 to 140 pounds during those eight months and in the last month she lost 5 pounds because of the hot weather and a low-salt diet. On September 17th, she went into labor and was admitted to the second floor of the Kingsville Hospital, where the white and Hispanic people were cared for. The first floor was for the blacks. I sat with her during labor, which was intense and lasted six hours, but she refused to take any pain medication. Then I assisted Dr. Walling in the delivery room because he only had one nurse, who had not worked in a delivery room for a long time. Martha Sue was born by essentially natural childbirth and only a saddle block, weighing 5 pounds 12 ounces, 19½ inches long. She cried when her head and shoulders were out of the birth canal and quickly turned pink. She was the first grandchild for my parents. Woody tried to nurse the baby but her breasts were engorged and Martha Sue did not know how to latch on to the areola and nipple. We were helped by one of the older nurses, who brought in a nipple shield, which fits over the breast and has a standard rubber nipple. With this, Martha Sue began to feed well but continued to require the nipple shield throughout the next four months. We were incredibly thrilled to have this first baby. She was alert and responsive but looked to us to be so thin and delicate. We had no family to help or advise us. I found out that I had little practical knowledge about newborns. Woody had a lot of educational knowledge about children but little practical knowledge about newborns either. Our pediatrician, Dr. Walter Watson, did not want Woody to nurse the baby. He kept telling us that she would gain weight faster if we put her on a formula and started baby foods. He finally convinced Woody to stop nursing at the end of four months but Martha did not gain any faster.

The other addition to our family was a cat named Minnie, the first of a long line of cats which we have had throughout our married life. Kittens were brought to us in a box by some children and Woody chose the little white kitten with one green eye and one blue eye. Minnie became very devoted to the new baby and

Martha Sue was fascinated with her. Minnie never "stole the breath" from the baby as the Navy wives warned us.

In July, I began to see patients come to sick call, almost all servicemen, with a syndrome of high fever, chills, prostration, no rash, a low white count and lung infiltrations on X-ray. This illness lasted about five days and was followed by a good deal of fatigue. I thought that these people had viral pneumonia and did not treat them with antibiotics. In November and December when the weather became cooler, the cases stopped coming. In June of the next year new cases reappeared.

I tried to save pilots who were involved in crash landings. One of my first was a pilot who tried to turn too sharply as he came about to land at South Field and crashed his plane. I got to him quickly and pulled him out of the plane. He was bleeding massively from his nose and throat and had an open fracture of his frontal bone with protruding brain. I gave him intravenous saline and put down an endotracheal tube to keep his airway open, and we airlifted him to the naval hospital in Corpus Christi. On the way, I continued to suction the blood out of his throat with my mouth because we had no suction apparatus, while I held a dressing over the protruding brain. He died shortly after we arrived at the naval hospital. The X-ray showed that he had a basal skull fracture which caused his bleeding. This was a horrifying experience for me. Most of my dying patients in Boston had been elderly, or if young had been known to have a terminal illness. I had not seen healthy young men with their lives ahead of them suddenly smashed to pieces. I began to have bad dreams and these crash scenes recurred as "flashbacks."

In my next crash experience I went out in the helicopter to find a pilot who was coming back to the base when his jet engine stopped functioning, a so-called "flame out." He was told to eject from the plane. We found the crash site but the pilot was buried in the ground still strapped in his seat. The canopy and the seat ejected but he must have been rendered unconscious and did not release himself from the seat or deploy his parachute. The third crash was also a flame-out and again the man was told to eject but did not. He ended up landing on an open field but unfortunately coasted into a patch of mesquite trees. I found him sitting in the seat of the plane with the canopy off and his helmet missing. With the help of the helicopter pilot, I carefully lifted him out and found that he was dead because of head injuries from the tree branches. In the subsequent investigation, the board of inquiry found out that the 38mm cannon shell that was used to propel the ejection seat out of his plane was a dud. They then checked all planes with ejection seats and found that many of the planes had 38mm shells that were old and nonfunctional. In other words, the men in those planes were flying in a coffin. A pilot cannot crawl out of a jet plane at 200 to 300 miles per hour. This scandal led to the appointment of a new commanding officer for our base. He was known in the Navy as a troubleshooter and in no time he began to whip the place into shape.

My fourth remarkable crash experience occurred when a student pilot was practicing dive-bombing. His instructor warned him that he was pulling out of the dive too sharply, "pulling too many Gs" (times gravity). As he came up to a level position, he looked out and saw both wings fall off the plane. The plane then began to dive backwards toward the ground, tail first, and made a long glide into the ground with the pilot still in the seat. The plane fell into pieces but the cockpit stayed intact with the pilot still belted in. A field worker came over, helped him out of the plane and covered the pilot with his open map to shield him from the sun. We flew 120 miles to the site in our slow Sikorsky helicopter carrying a black bag containing some intravenous saline, morphine, and bandages. I found the pilot alive, covered with deep lacerations, and in severe pain which I relieved with morphine. The old rule of trauma is "splint them where they lie," so I used pieces off the plane and branches from the mesquite bushes and wrapped him in the positions in which his limbs were found, using every article of bandage and clothing we had to pad him. Then we hung him in a rack underneath the helicopter. I plugged in intravenous saline and we set off for the naval hospital in Corpus Christi. When we arrived, we took him immediately to X-ray and to everyone's surprise he had no fractures. He then was taken to the operating room and his lacerations were closed. Within a few weeks, he was sent back to our base to finish his training. He lodged a complaint against me because of the crude and primitive splints which I had used. The Sikorsky Helicopter Company gave me a medal for "saving a pilot with their helicopter." This pilot finished his training and was given leave to go home to Chicago before reporting to California for carrier landings. He drove a fast sport car and was killed in a collision driving home just outside of Chicago. This sad outcome was so ironic because he was the only pilot that survived a crash that I attended.

The last crash I will describe resulted in the death of a student and his instructor, a Marine captain. One of the instructor's student pilots was a Naval Academy graduate who had become a close friend of this captain and his family. He was in the Officer's Club the following afternoon drinking and began to cry about the loss of his instructor. Other pilots began to laugh at him and implied that he was too close to his friend, perhaps in a homosexual relationship. The student became enraged and warned the others that they would be sorry if they kept up the ridicule. He ran to his room and came back with two pearl-handled revolvers. He threatened to shoot the scoffers and backed them up against the bar. Someone called a Marine guard but the student got the drop on him and disarmed him. Then someone called Commander X, the executive officer of the base, who tried to convince the student to lay down his guns, but ended up against the bar with the rest. Finally someone called the dispensary, where I was on duty, and told the whole story. I filled a syringe with 100 mg of chlorpromazine, a potent tranquilizer, and asked Langham, my smartest and coolest corpsman, to come with me and bring a straitjacket. We entered the side door of the club and I walked up the man with the guns pointing at me while Langham circled around behind him. He said to me, "Who the hell are you?" I told him that I was the doctor, that he had gone crazy and that I was going to take him to the hospital. I shoved the needle into his shoulder muscle right through his shirt and injected the full dose of drug. Langham reached around from behind and took both revolvers from his hands. Then we placed the straitjacket over his head and strapped his arms to his sides. He offered no resistance as we marched him to the ambulance and drove him to the naval hospital. I telephoned the psychiatrist on duty and told him the story. Langham returned in the ambulance and reported that the student became somnolent and was carried into the hospital. To my amazement he was back at our base two days later along with a note from the psychiatrist saying that the man showed no psychotic ideas or behavior when he woke up from the chlorpromazine and could return to duty. He did not record the real reasons for the student's hospital admission because it might ruin the career of an Academy graduate, The man was never disciplined, never spoke to me and graduated from the flight program.

Many more crashes occurred that required me to go to the rescue which I will not describe. My bad dreams became more frequent after these experiences and I realize now that I was suffering from a form of post-traumatic stress disorder. Finally, we got some regulation splints to carry in the helicopter but we never did get radios that allowed us to communicate with the planes in the air. These were old helicopters that had been discontinued in Korea and had an open door on one side. A doctor at Corpus Christi Naval Air Station drowned when this model helicopter crashed into the Gulf of Mexico and he was trapped in the wreckage. The maintenance person who took care of our helicopter was an enlisted man who was often in trouble and often at sick call for various complaints. On one New Year's Eve, he came in dead drunk, having been beaten up in a fight with the shore patrol. I left the New Year's Eve party at the officer's club and spent hours sewing up the lacerations of his scalp without local anesthesia. My faith in his ability to maintain our helicopter was permanently shaken and I feared for my life every time I flew in it.

I finally got caught by the rule that all obstetric cases needing delivery had to get to Corpus Christi Naval Hospital. An officer's wife went into rapid labor and came into the dispensary and we all agreed she would never make it to the naval hospital. The corpsman did not want to deliver her in the ambulance. I set her up in stirrups in the operating room and examined her. The baby's head was low in the birth canal and ready to be delivered. Unfortunately, the presentation was posterior, not left occiput anterior, which is the proper position for delivering a baby. I had no forceps so I could not turn the baby's head. I called our friendly Kingsville obstetrician, Dr. Walling, for help. We drove the mother to the hospital in town, he turned the baby's head and in two minutes she was delivered and everybody did well. I never had to attempt another delivery in the dispensary.

Stan Wiener gave us notice that his tour of duty was up and left to go back to Denver to his cardiology training and to have his daughter's cleft palate repaired. Our new flight surgeon was Robert Hoover. He had a wonderful family, consisting of his wife, Freda, and three boys, John, Billy and Freddy. Billy in particular became a favorite of my daughter Martha. Bob was a sensible and well-trained general practitioner and the pilots loved him. Our next addition was Vercel Fuglestad, a man from Minnesota who had two years of surgical training. His wife, Marsha, was expecting her first baby. Vercel was a great help because he took over the "minor surgery" and some of the orthopedics that I had struggled with. The next addition was John Eisenlohr, a surgical intern from Southwestern Medical Center in Dallas, who had already obtained an ophthalmology residency at Johns Hopkins Hospital. Finally, Dr. Merwin Dieckman showed up. He was from Iowa Medical School and had worked one year as a general practitioner. His wife, Betty, delivered twins shortly after their arrival in Kingsville. One was a normal girl and the other a tiny boy with a very small head, who was profoundly retarded because his placenta was too small and he was inadequately nourished in the womb. Shortly after the boy, David, was born he developed pneumonia. John Eisenlohr and I tried to convince Merwin not to give him any antibiotics but to let him die a natural death. However, Merwin and his wife insisted on treating him and this boy then lived for nineteen years in a state no more mature than that of a three-month-old baby.

My life was now more pleasant because I was only on duty every fourth night and fourth weekend and was home at noon after I had night duty. I went to crashes only every fourth call. We now lived in town on Alice Street in a house with a fenced back yard. Minnie died crossing a road but our life with cats continued when my former medical school roommate sent us a male and a female Siamese cat because his wife became allergic to cats. We lived next to Texas College of Agriculture and Industry, which meant that we had accessible baby-sitters. Both Woody and I became members of bowling teams. Ours consisted of the recently promoted Captain N, John Eisenlohr, myself and an enlisted man who was a 200-average bowler, a "ringer" on our doctors' team. Unfortunately, we came to work one morning and found him being arrested by the shore patrol because he was caught in bed with a young recruit. The Navy considers homosexual activity a fearful crime and everybody panics and rushes these people off into the brig. The Captain was furious. He said he could not understand why this man behaved so badly and showed "no loyalty or gratitude after being allowed to bowl on our team".

In the summer of 1955, the mysterious febrile illness among the enlisted men and pilots returned with a vengeance. This time, I collected blood at the beginning of the illness and then three weeks later. I sent the serum samples off to Washington, D.C., to Walter Reed Army Hospital. I asked them to test for antibodies to many pulmonary infections, viral and bacterial. To my great surprise, everything came back negative except for rising titers of antibodies to Q fever (Q stands for query). This is an illness caused by a rickettsial organism called *Coxiella burnetii*. It is an intracellular parasite and a member of a family of rickettsia that also cause Rocky Mountain spotted fever and typhus. Q fever is marked by high fever, chills, malaise, dry cough and pneumonia as seen in my patients. It can also involve the liver and heart valves, but fortunately this did not occur in my previously healthy men. Once I knew the cause of this syndrome I treated the patients with tetracycline, which shortened the duration of the acute illness from 5-8 days to 3-5 days and reduced the post-illness fatigue. I drove my car to San Antonio, Texas, to Brooke Army Medical Center to use their library. There, I reviewed all the published literature about Q fever. I collected serum from the men who had had the syndrome the previous summer and had them tested for antibodies to Q fever. Most of them still had a significant titer of antibodies. My total number of cases was 33. I wrote a medical article to report what I called "Endemic Q fever in South Texas." It was published in the *Armed Forces Medical Journal* in October of 1956. The reason that the cases were all between July and December each year is that the rickettsial infectious particles were spread by ticks to cattle. The dried tick bodies in the soil or on cattle hides contained Q fever rickettsia resistant to drying and were spread in the dust storms each summer and fall. The portal of entry in humans was through the lungs by inhalation. It is really a disease of cows and other animals; humans are an accidental second host. Residents of south

Texas are often infected early in life but newly arrived Navy personnel are not immune and are highly susceptible to infection.

In January of 1956, a terrible new disease came to our base. Poliomyelitis entered the United States from Mexico across the Rio Grande border that year and we began to have cases in children and adults in January and February. The men and their dependents went into a panic because of fear of this disease. We had a limited supply of immune gamma-globulin to prevent the disease so we gave it only to pregnant women and children, who are most susceptible. An aviator, a Captain in the Marine Corps, came to see Captain N and insisted on getting gamma-globulin because a polio case had occurred in his part of the housing compound. Despite our rule, the captain gave in and administered gamma-globulin to him. This exception led to demands by other pilots and their wives for the globulin. None of the doctors, nurses or medical corpsmen was treated.

Our baby, Martha Sue, and my wife, Woody, who was now pregnant again, received the gamma-globulin. Woody's bowling team came to our house for dessert and coffee and one of the women who was helping wash up the dishes told my wife that she was feeling terrible. She had a headache and felt feverish. During that night, she developed bulbar polio, had difficulty breathing and swallowing and became paralyzed in her lower extremities. We took her by ambulance, supporting her breathing, to the naval hospital at Corpus Christi. I did not know what happened to her until eight months later when I was a resident rotating through the Boston Lying-In Hospital. A woman came in for delivery who was paralyzed in her lower extremities. She was my wife's bowling partner. Things got so bad in Kingsville that every child who came into the dispensary with a minor illness underwent a lumbar puncture. We found a number of children who had cells in their spinal fluid and had nonparalytic or mildly paralytic polio. Unfortunately, a number of them developed significant paralysis. The disease finally burned out in south Texas by the end of the spring. Polio spread across the country and caused numerous deaths and paralyses. It was the last of the great polio epidemics because the Salk polio vaccine was released that very year.

One last case I will describe was at first ominous and eventually humorous. I was on duty when someone called from town to report that an enlisted man and his wife got into a fight and she shot him in the heart with a 22-caliber pistol. He was still alive so we rushed to his house by ambulance and found that he had an entrance wound over his heart but no exit wound and he had normal vital signs. His wife was crying loudly and begging his forgiveness. We took him to the dispensary and took a chest X-ray. No bullet could be seen. An abdominal film showed the bullet in his left buttock. We concluded that the bullet hit a rib over his left front chest, followed the groove of the rib around to the back and then down into his left gluteal muscle. It never entered his chest cavity. After the bullet was removed he and his wife made up and she promised never to shoot him again.

I want to pay tribute to the doctors who worked with me at Kingsville. We were either drafted into the Navy or volunteered after we were about to be drafted. John Eisenlohr was so bright and competent. A woman brought in a baby who was gray in color and not breathing. John quickly took forceps, reached down the baby's throat, felt a foreign body and pulled it out. A pacifier had become wedged into its trachea so it could not breathe. Astoundingly, in spite of lacking oxygen so long, this baby recovered and functioned normally. John went on to the Wilmer Eye Institute at Johns Hopkins, where he rose to be chief resident and then went back to practice ophthalmology in Dallas. We have stayed in touch all these years. Bob Hoover finished his tour of duty and went to Florida to do family practice. Merwin Dieckman went to do family practice in Tennessee. Vercel Fuglestad took a challenge from some of the pilots that he could not pass their ground school, so he enrolled and passed with flying colors. They then put him in a plane with an instructor. He took off and landed the plane, based on his ground school training. In the summer of 1955, he became ill and an X-ray showed that he had cystic lesions in his upper lobe, which I thought might be tuberculosis. We sent him to St. Albans Naval Hospital on Long Island and they did a resection of the upper lobe of his lung, which showed not TB, but coccidioidomycosis, a common fungal disease of south Texas. It is usually a self-limited illness in healthy young people. I began to see more cases come in after this experience. I kept and observed them and did not transfer them for surgery. After Vercel left the Navy, he went back to Minnesota to finish his surgical training and practiced surgery there for many years. He became a skilled pilot and flew planes all over the United States and on mission trips to Africa.

We had a frightening episode concerning our baby daughter, Martha Sue. At four months of age, our pediatrician told us that she had an abnormally small head, what he called "microcephaly," and predicted that she would be mentally retarded. This prognosis was impossible for us to believe because her growth and development up to that time had been normal. It was true that her head was smaller than 95 percent of babies her age. In order to get a second opinion, I called Baylor Medical Center in Houston and got an appointment with the Department of Pediatrics for a workup on a Saturday morning. The chief of pediatrics was a man named Russell Blattner, a nationally prominent pediatrician. He had an excellent staff of doctors who put Martha Sue in one day through a complete evaluation of her cognitive functions, such as they are in a 4-month-old baby. Then he told us that she was normal and her small head size was at the end of the normal curve, to our great relief. He asked if anybody in our families had a small head. Woody's parents had worried because her head was small and other members of her family had small heads. When he read her maiden name, Lagemann, he said "Could you by any chance be related to a 'Fritz' Lagemann who sang in the Glee Club with me at the University of Missouri?" This was indeed Woody's father, Alfred Frederick Lagemann, nicknamed Fritz by his college friends. Thirty years later on a trip to Houston I telephoned him and told him that his evaluation of that baby was accurate. Martha went on to grow and develop normally. She became a skilled gymnast, graduated Phi Beta Kappa from Oberlin College with a double major in Russian and German, received an MA in Slavic languages from Indiana University and was currently employed at Radio Free Europe/Radio Liberty in Munich as an editor and researcher. He was greatly pleased to get such a positive follow-up of his judgment.

We had decided around Christmas of 1955 that we wanted to have another baby and fortunately had no problem conceiving. Unfortunately, we got into a recurrent problem that went back to Martha Sue's pregnancy. Because of bleeding in the first three weeks and a history of two miscarriages, her obstetrician at the Boston Lying-In Hospital, a Harvard hospital, put Woody on a drug called diethyl stilbestrol, or DES, which was supposed to prevent miscarriages. I did not know that a study had already been done at Harvard showing that DES was not effective in this regard. Everybody at the Lying-In Hospital believed in it however. Woody took large doses of DES until Martha Sue was born. Again with this second pregnancy she began to spot at three weeks. Dr. Walling became concerned and said we had better try DES again since it seemed to help the first time. Now I believe that this was probably normal implantation bleeding. So Woody took DES through the second pregnancy, up to a few weeks before delivery. Unfortunately, this drug causes a disease in female children marked by benign tumors and adhesions in the vagina, so-called vaginal adenosis, and rarely other cancers, as in the case of our second child, who had cancer of the cervix in situ at the age of 22. Thankfully this was cured at Sloan Kettering Hospital in New York City by conization of the cervix. The complications from DES therapy eventually led to thousands of lawsuits against the drug companies that made this agent.

We drove to Boston in June 1956 for the wedding of my sister, Suzanne, to Richard Gordon Hosford, a graduate of Harvard Medical School in the Class of 1957. Woody moved into the housing project near the Brigham with my medical school classmate John Whitcomb and his wife, Dorothy, both Oberlin classmates, and their two babies and used it as a base to go house hunting. I had to fly back to Kingsville to be discharged on June 30th. While I was there I became quite anxious about going out on any more helicopter flights; nevertheless two more helicopter flights were required of me. I left Captain N to deal with the Navy's concerns about this "epidemic" of Q fever about which he knew nothing. Finally, I was discharged from the Navy and left July 1st to fly to Boston to begin my junior residency at the Peter Bent Brigham Hospital.

5

Junior Residency

◆

1956–1957

I returned from the Navy on July 1, 1956, to begin my junior assistant residency at the Peter Bent Brigham Hospital. Because I was two years older than the interns who had gone directly into the junior residency and because of my Navy experience, Dr. Thorn and Dr. Eugene Eppinger, his house staff coordinator, assigned me to begin on the semiprivate ward, F-Second, which was the most difficult assignment for the year's rotation. My new intern was a man named Martin Liebowitz, a graduate of NYU Medical School. I was so fortunate to begin my residency with him. Martin is a wonderful human being and, in addition, he was a quick learner and a hard worker and he had a warm personality when relating to patients. We formed a good partnership and got off to a great start together. We have remained friends ever since that time. He later became a professor at the State University of New York at Stony Brook and chief of the medical service at their VA Hospital. We saw each other regularly when I later became chief of the medical service at the VA Hospital in Indianapolis. Our most memorable patient was a young man with a stroke, which we proved came from a septic embolus originating on a coarctation of the aorta; antibiotics and aortic surgery cured him.

After this first rotation in August, I moved over to E-Second, where I had a new intern who was the opposite of Dr. Liebowitz. This man was a graduate of Harvard Medical School and seemed to lack the milk of human kindness necessary for a doctor. He had difficulty getting along with patients because he argued with them and lectured them rather than working with them. He was also poor at doing procedures. He ruined so many patients' veins drawing blood and putting in intravenous feedings that a delegation of patients came to me to declare they were going on strike against him and would not let him do any more procedures on them. Therefore, I took him into the doctor's workroom with a handful of syringes and needles. We sat down opposite each other and I taught him the technique of venipuncture that Dr. Carl Walter, one of the surgeons at the Brigham, had taught me. I stuck him in his arm vein to show him how to do it and then I had him stick me. He messed it up. I then stuck him again and showed him, "do it this way." He stuck me and messed it up. I stuck him and we continued this until he finally learned how to do it properly. Then we walked around the ward and apologized to the patients. I told them that they would find his technique had now improved and that he would get along with them better. They agreed to let him be their doctor again and he finally finished out the month with moderate success.

Before I began the rotation Woody had been living with our classmates, John and Dotty Whitcomb, looking at housing ads and going out every day with Martha Sue in the general area around the Brigham looking for an apartment that we could afford. Under the GI Bill, I was going to receive $300 a month and the Brigham was going to pay me the great sum of $50 a month. Thus we were limited in how much a month we could pay for housing. We tried to get an apartment at the Mission Hill Housing Project across from the Brigham. This was for people whose income was quite low. We qualified, so I asked for a ground-floor apartment because Woody was pregnant. The only apartment they would offer us was one on the third floor. I was advised by the man who ran the drugstore on the corner, Joe Sparr, that we could not get a good apartment in the Housing Project unless we left a contribution on the seat of the chair after the interview. So I asked the assignment man one more time to please give us a ground-floor apartment. I left $50 under a newspaper and walked out. We never did get the apartment even though we knew there were first-floor ones available. Woody continued searching and finally found an apartment in Belmont that looked satisfactory and only cost $75 a month. The great thing about this flat was its location, just across the street from a wonderful playground. In order to help pay the costs of the apartment and of our living expenses during that year I borrowed $800 from my father and eventually paid it back. Martha Sue was happy to have playmates who lived in our apartment building and in the surrounding houses and to have a playground just across the street.

Woody's pregnancy had gone well and she was due on September 20th. I took my vacation during that week so I could take care of Martha Sue while she had the baby and later when she was home with the new baby. However, her pregnancy continued until September 27th, when she finally went into labor. She told her obstetrician at the Boston Lying-In Hospital that she did not want pain medications or scopolamine or general anesthesia during her delivery, which was the standard routine at the Boston Lying-In. Her doctor was unhappy about having to deliver a natural childbirth because he was not used to this experience. The baby came down with the head posterior, not in the normal anterior position, and did not enter the birth canal, so-called high transverse arrest. The doctor did not attempt external version, a procedure for turning the baby from the outside of the abdomen in between contractions. Then, without anesthesia he went ahead and did a mid-forceps delivery, reaching up into the uterus, putting the forceps on the baby's head, pulling it down, turning it to the anterior position and bringing it out. The baby girl was born with a rather molded and misshapen head and was quite lethargic. It took her 48 hours to awaken fully and begin to nurse. Jennifer, as we named her, was a wonderful baby but we soon noted that she did not have normal movements of her left leg and hand. The hand was flaccid and she dragged her leg when she began crawling. We finally found a neurologist who made the diagnosis of cerebral palsy, fortunately mild. Eventually she recovered normal use of her left arm, hand and leg. I have never forgiven this obstetrician for mismanaging Jennifer's delivery. Martha Sue, however, was so excited and happy about her new sister. She loved her completely from the moment she met her and never showed jealousy. Her first question was, "When can she play with me?"

My next rotation was a strange one, a patchwork rotation during September and October of 1956. First of all I worked in the outpatient admitting room, in a small office where I dealt with the patients who walked in to be seen. It was my job to triage them to the emergency ward, admit them to the hospital, schedule a clinic appointment or treat them and send them home. It was like being back in Navy sick call but I was seeing 80 to 100 patients a day and they were much sicker than the young people in the Navy.

We were asked to supervise the intern in the emergency ward who was on duty during the day. I recall being asked to see a 19-year-old girl who had shot herself in the temple with a 22-caliber rifle in a suicide attempt. The bullet passed through her head at eye level and severed her optic nerves, rendering her blind but not killing her. We learned that she was single and had become pregnant by her boyfriend, who abandoned her. She was too ashamed to tell her parents so she decided to kill herself with her father's rifle. I know she recovered from the injury but never heard what became of her.

In the evenings, we went to the heart station and read the electrocardiograms (EKGs) that had been taken all over the hospital during that day. Then in the early morning we presented our EKG readings to the staff cardiologist, who criticized our interpretations and changed them to make a final report. The two main electrocardiographers were Harold Levine and Bernard Lown. These men were highly competent in this specialty and also good cardiologists. In these two months I read basic texts on electrocardiography and learned by practice to be competent in reading electrocardiograms. I always have been able to read EKGs in the heat of emergencies from then on.

I also recall that we continued to work in our own medical clinic one day a week. This was a disappointment as far as a learning experience because there was nobody who was supervising us and no one to discuss our cases with. The patients waited interminably to see the doctors. Every other night we covered the emergency ward and admitted patients to the wards that were not covered by a senior resident. This experience was most enjoyable because we could help interns learn to do the job in the emergency ward. We also continued to work one evening in the syphilis clinic.

One of the more interesting parts of this rotation was serving as a consultant at the Boston Lying-In Hospital. One day a week we worked in a clinic in which women with medical diseases complicating their pregnancies were seen and managed. This clinic was started by Dr. C. Sydney Burwell, our professor at the Brigham, and was staffed by his associate, Dr. James Metcalfe, who had been trained as a resident at the Brigham and then spent time in physiology learning about pregnancy. Based on their experience at the Boston Lying-In, Jim and Dr. Burwell wrote the definitive book on the care of medical complications of pregnancy. We were also called as consultants to go to the Lying-In to see patients who were admitted with medical problems and then we presented these patients to Dr. Metcalfe. I learned a great deal from this experience. One patient raised serious ethical considerations long before these problems were being discussed. The woman had Hodgkin's disease, a cancer of the lymphocytes, and was undergoing chemotherapy when she was found to be pregnant. The doctors finished the chemotherapy and advised her to have an abortion because the baby had been exposed to these dangerous chemotherapy drugs at an early stage of its development. However, she was a strict Catholic and refused to have an abortion and insisted in carrying on the pregnancy. To our amazement, she had a normal baby.

One of the main problems in the clinic was patients with heart disease. Women with rheumatic heart disease are particularly prone to develop narrowing of their mitral valve, where the blood flows from the lungs into the left side of the heart before it is pumped out to the rest of the body. The narrow mitral valve causes a pressure rise in the blood vessels of the lungs and this leads to fluid in the lungs, so-called pulmonary edema. As the pregnancy progresses their blood volume increases and the pressure rises higher in the lung blood vessels. These women were extremely brittle and suddenly could go into pulmonary edema. They were difficult to manage medically and many of them died during their pregnancy or an emergency abortion had to be done to get them out of trouble. At the Peter Bent Brigham, Dr. Dwight Harken, the pioneer cardiac surgeon, was doing a procedure called mitral valvuloplasty in which he opened up the chest, stuck his forefinger into the upper chamber of the heart (the left atrium) down through the mitral valve and fractured the calcium and scar tissue with his finger, opening up the mitral valve. He decided to take women who looked like they weren't going to make it through their pregnancy and did a mitral valvuloplasty. To our amazement, he was able to do this successfully without causing premature labor and the loss of the fetus. After the finger fracture of the mitral valve, these women improved markedly and got through their pregnancy without further trouble. It was during this rotation at the Boston Lying-In that I met again the Navy wife who had come down with polio nine months before in Kingsville, Texas. She successfully delivered a baby even though she was paralyzed from the waist down.

My next rotation lasted four months at the West Roxbury VA Hospital, which was affiliated with the Brigham. We staffed two large wards with forty patients on each. A senior resident supervised each ward and two junior residents. The West Roxbury VA Hospital at that time was not an up-to-date organization. For example, we could get no emergency electrolyte measurements or blood sugars during the night because the laboratory was closed. This made it extremely difficult to take care of diabetic ketoacidosis or dehydration cases. The chief of the medical service, Dr. T. A. Warthin, was a former military man who had some training in gastroenterology. He was particularly concerned that things look right even if they were not and when something went wrong his major concern was whom he would blame. We had a mantra that resulted from this behavior: "T.A. is the D.A. of the VA."

The rule of the VA in those days was that the hospital beds had to be kept full at all times, because they were paid by the government on the basis of patients in beds. So if we discharged ten patients in one day, ten more patients would be admitted the same day, whether they needed to come in to the hospital or not. The admitting service was under the control of career VA doctors who knew the system and were not concerned about the actual needs of the patients for admission. We residents covered the night admissions, which was a blessing for them and for us. The VA had good surgical staffing furnished by the Brigham. The other fault of the system in those days was that there was no outpatient clinic care unless the veteran was service-connected which meant that he went downtown in

Boston to a clinic on Court Street. If he was not service-connected the VA hospital gave him a one-week supply of medications, prescriptions for more, and no outpatient appointment and discharged him. The veterans, who were usually poor, ran out of medicines, rarely refilled their prescriptions and came back into the hospital within a few weeks with the same problem they had been treated for before. Many patients were very ill but a few patients did not need to be in the hospital. They talked the admitting doctors into being admitted so they could spend the summer in Boston. Later, they would go to Arizona or Florida to spend the winter in another VA hospital.

The West Roxbury patients presented us with an amazing spectrum of diseases and we learned a great deal. One interesting patient I recall was being followed by Dr. Warthin for a rare and usually fatal condition called Whipple's disease. It was a disease that involved all of the organs of the body but in particular the small bowel and caused diarrhea, weight loss and poor absorption of food. He came into the hospital for one of his recurrent admissions and while there he suddenly went into remission and regained almost complete health. Dr. Warthin asked me to review his chart and try to find out what we had done on this admission that was different from previous admissions that could have led to his amazing improvement. The only things that were different were that he had received two transfusions of fresh blood and had a course of penicillin treatment for a respiratory infection. Dr. Warthin decided that it must have been the fresh blood transfusions and never followed up on the possibility that it might have been the antibiotic. Neither of us knew that in 1952, a Dr. Paulley had reported a complete remission of Whipple's Disease after a course of another antibiotic, chloramphenicol. So we missed a chance to report an important finding to the medical literature. The intestinal biopsies and the biopsies of lymph nodes in the these patients showed large cells called macrophages packed with red staining material (staining with periodic acid Schiff reagent) and even under light microscopy it looked like there were bacteria within these cells. Later, when electron microscopy became available, we could see that there were bacterial rods in the cells of patients with Whipple's disease. Finally with great difficulty these organisms were cultured, found to be a species of *actinobacter* and given the name *Tropheryma whippli*. It is now clear that this disease responds to many antibiotics and is no longer a fatal disease.

I had an unfortunate patient named Chester who kept being admitted. He had a rare blood condition called myeloid metaplasia. In his case I found out that it resulted from being exposed to benzene on a job, for which he should have received, but did not receive, compensation. As often occurs the myeloid metaplasia changed over into acute myeloid leukemia and Chester was told that he would have to undergo powerful and often unsuccessful chemotherapy. He became depressed and jumped from the sixth-floor bathroom window onto the concrete below, committing suicide. This caused a major upset on the medical service. Two days later, a patient with severe heart failure and depression pried open the window of his room, tied some sheets to his bed, crawled out down the sheets and dropped six floors into the snow and was found dead in the morning. Later, a third patient committed suicide. Dr. Warthin was extremely agitated because people came from the main VA office to investigate what was happening on his medical service. He had the problem of trying to assign blame for the lack of patient supervision and the lack of suicide preventive measures while excusing himself of responsibility.

During that winter, just after Christmas, we had an enormous snowfall in Boston and the city was paralyzed. The hospital lost all power. We had an emergency generator in the hospital but the electrician who had the only key to turn it on lived on the other side of the city. The police finally found a four-wheeled vehicle which could get through the snow and brought him to the hospital. In the intervening eight hours before he arrived we went down to the spinal cord injury ward and hand pumped the "iron lung" machines of the patients who were unable to breathe and were supported by their iron lungs.

John Harter, my intern partner from the Brigham, was also my partner as a junior resident. We had a senior resident named Joseph Shipp who was a strict, obsessive and humorless type doctor, who was always correcting us and writing notes in our charts in green ink. John Harter absolutely abhorred him. They argued every day while we made rounds. Joseph told me, "That month with John Harter was the worst experience of my training years." The last two months our senior resident was Tom Newcomb, a quiet, intelligent, laid-back type who got along with everybody and let the junior residents carry the ball. Tom went on to become head of the Research Service of the VA in Central Office in Washington, DC.

The nurses at the VA had been there for years and were quite impervious to changing what they did or learning new approaches. The head nurse on our ward missed my order to stop the three daily doses of digoxin which we used to "load" a patient to get him out of heart failure. I changed the order to one tablet a day but the nurses continued to give him three a day and he died of digitalis intoxication because of an arrhythmia. In the investigation that followed, the head nurse's mistake was found and yet she never received a reprimand nor were procedures changed to prevent such errors in the future.

One of the good things about the VA was that we had wonderful attending physicians and consultants who came not only from the Brigham but from other hospitals all over Boston. Our neurology consultant was Dr. Joseph Foley from Boston City Hospital, one of the best neurologists in town. I received a consultation from the resident on the genitourinary ward about a patient there who had a fever. He told me that as part of his fever workup he did a spinal tap and sent the spinal fluid to the laboratory. They called back to say that the spinal fluid was loaded with acid-fast bacilli like those of tuberculosis but there were no white blood cells in the spinal fluid. I went to see the patient, who did not look ill, and I called Dr. Foley and told him the story. He said, "Phil, that patient would have to be dead not to have a cellular response to tubercle bacilli in his spinal fluid. Something is wrong with this specimen. Go back and talk to the GU resident and find out what happened before and after the spinal tap". When I discussed it with him, the young surgeon told me that before he did the spinal tap, he had catheterized the patient to get a urine specimen for culture and analysis. He wore the same pair of gloves during the catheterization and during the spinal tap. The patient had not been circumcised and when the surgeon pulled back his foreskin, underneath was a cheesy white collection loaded with *Mycobacterium smegmatis,* a bacterium which is acid-fast like tuberculosis bacteria when stained in the laboratory. It is a harmless and nonpathogenic bacteria but looked just like tubercle bacilli. This is how he had contaminated the normal spinal fluid with these bacteria and that is why there were no white cells in the spinal fluid. When I called Dr. Foley to tell him the rest of the story, he roared with laughter and added the story to his repertoire of humorous disease consultations.

Our VA experience was greatly appreciated by Brigham residents, in spite of the faults of the hospital system, because the veterans needed our help and liked their doctors. We were able to keep them for weeks to months to stabilize or rehabilitate them and to care for them until they either reached time for discharge or died. There was no hurry in those days to discharge patients. I cared for one middle-aged man who came in with a mild stroke leading to partial paralysis of the left arm and leg. We treated his high blood pressure, which was the background for the stroke, and put him through two months of rehabilitation so when he left he was able to walk with a splint on his leg but could not use the left arm. He went back to his job. Shortly thereafter, I received a call from the Internal Revenue Service who told me that they were not going to allow my GI Bill payments to be tax exempt because they did not consider training as a medical resident as "going to school." They asked me to come to the IRS office to discuss it with them. They assigned me to a man sitting at a desk and when he looked up he said, "Dr. Snodgrass, what are you doing here?" It was my patient who had had the stroke and he was back working at the IRS even though he could only use his right arm. Needless to say this grateful patient made sure that I got tax exemption on my GI Bill payments.

We all appreciated the fact that we could get advice from almost any doctor in Boston if needed for our patients at the VA. For example, among our consultants who came out to discuss difficult patient were Franz Ingelfinger, the famous gastroenterologist; Joseph Foley, the neurologist from Boston City; Charles Davidson, the liver expert from Boston City Hospital; and the Chief of Medicine at Boston City, Dr. William B. Castle, who had isolated intrinsic factor in pernicious anemia. One of our best teachers was Dr. Louis Weinstein, the infectious disease expert from Boston University. By using these experts, we were able to make up for deficiencies in our Brigham training. At that time, there were no Brigham rotations, only consultations, in rheumatology, infectious disease, or neurology, although they were subsequently developed. Looking back on my VA experience I can honestly say that I enjoyed the patient care but learned to dislike the old VA system.

My last rotation in the spring was at the Deaconess Hospital, in particular, the Joslin Clinic service at the Deaconess. Elliott Joslin had founded the clinic to take care of diabetics before insulin had been discovered. Then the only treatment for these people was a high-fat diet, the so-called ketogenic diet, to try to keep them out of diabetic coma. Dr. Joslin had been one of the first in the country to receive insulin from Eli Lilly Company. He treated George Richards Minot, the famous hematologist at Boston City Hospital, and saved his life so that he could go on and discover the liver cure for pernicious anemia. Dr. Joslin kept his records all those years on 5 x 8 inch cards and wrote his notes in a tiny neat hand. I went back and read some of the original cards in his files about the famous patients that he had treated. He believed that frequent doses of regular insulin before meals or long-acting insulin combined with regular insulin plus strict dietary control and regular exercise would help regulate what we call Type I diabetes, a program we use today. His patients were expected to weigh all their food. This Type I diabetes occurs early in life and is an autoimmune disease and is associated with no insulin in the system. Type II diabetes, which we called adult onset, is associated with obesity and resistance to the insulin which is produced by the patient's pancreas. Dr. Joslin had very strong opinions but they were based on his anecdotal experience. He never carried out any controlled studies and neither did the other doctors at the Joslin Clinic. We use to tease him at morning report when we presented patients we had admitted during the night. I presented a patient from Brookline, Massachusetts, who developed diabetes in 1918 and survived until insulin came along and then for many years gave himself one injection in the morning of the longest-acting insulin, protamine zinc insulin. He never followed a diet. He was obese and on my examination showed no diabetic complications involving his eyes, kidneys, nerves or blood vessels. When I finished the presentation, Dr. Joslin said, "I don't think that history is true. I know for a fact that he often weighed his food." The Joslin staff all followed the policies of Elliott Joslin. It was just tradition. The most scientific member of the staff was a man named Alexander Marble and I latched on to him and stayed with him as much of the time that I could. He was the one who taught me how to control brittle Type I diabetics who were sent to the Joslin Clinic because no one else could control them. After his teaching and my managing many cases of diabetic ketoacidosis, I came out of this rotation confident that I could manage any diabetic patient.

The surgeons associated with the clinic were extremely good, particularly in the area of vascular disease, which was one of the plagues of long-term diabetics. The Deaconess Hospital excelled in its nursing, radiology and laboratory work, and was the polar opposite of the poor old VA hospital that we just left. One of the staff was a woman doctor, Priscilla White, whose primary interest was taking care of pregnant diabetics. These women had a tremendous drive to get pregnant and then to produce a live baby, although the miscarriage rate was high. Dr. White carefully controlled their blood sugar levels and often admitted them to the hospital for two to six months of bed rest, dietary control and frequent insulin doses. She was often able to get them a live baby. Subsequently new physicians came into the Joslin Clinic after the death of the old founder and the Clinic became a modern leader in studies of diabetic care, cause and management.

During the rotation in the spring, Warren Wacker asked me if I would come down and talk to Dr. Bert Vallee, who was the director of the Biophysics Research Laboratory in the basement of the Brigham. Warren was working as a research fellow in the laboratory and another resident whom I knew, Dr. David Ulmer, had joined the laboratory. I sat down with Bert and he asked me if I wanted to be a fellow for a period of training in biophysics and biochemistry. This had always been my major interest as a training experience for a career in academic medicine and I agreed to become a fellow in his lab. My next job was to apply for fellowship support. He recommended that I apply to The National Foundation which had formerly been the March of Dimes and researched and treated polio. Now it supported research in many areas of basic science and of growth and development. Dr. Vallee advised me that when I went to the interview in New York City, I should stress that fact that I had had no research experience of any importance and that I really needed serious research training, which in fact was true. So when I sat in front of this imposing group in the headquarters of The National Foundation in New York City and they quizzed me on my background I kept insisting that what I had done in college, medical school and residency was not acceptable research training but that I needed to work with Dr. Vallee and learn how to do first-class biochemical research. The committee accepted my application and I received the fellowship at the amazing stipend of $8,000 a year for two years, a major increase over the $3600 a year on the GI Bill I had been receiving during my junior residency. I completed my junior residency in June 1957 with a feeling that I had performed near the top of my resident class. The members of that class included an outstanding group of doctors who remained my friends for the rest of my life. I thought that I was about to embark on a period of research training which would help me enter a successful life in academic medicine.

6

Research Training

♦

1957–1959

I began my work in the Biophysics Research Laboratory on July 5, 1957, where I was assigned to work with one of the PhD analytical chemists, a man named Ralph Thiers. I was required to learn one of the basic analytical methods of the laboratory, which was to assay zinc using the dithizone colorimetric method. Dr. Bert L. Vallee was one of the world's experts on the role of zinc in biology and in particular of zinc firmly bound to enzymes. This trace-metal methodology was complex and particular. First of all, in order to avoid contamination, all of the glassware had to be metal-free, especially free of contaminating zinc. Therefore glassware was soaked in concentrated nitric and sulfuric acid over night and then rinsed six times in purified metal-free water. The fellows had to do the acid washing and rinsing themselves. A dishwasher was available to do this for the technicians. Then the glassware was dried in a special oven. If I wanted to analyze the zinc in a biological specimen, I would place the specimen in a metal-free silver or glass beaker, ash it in an oven overnight, dissolve the ash in metal-free hydrochloric acid, neutralize it and then extract the zinc using a zinc chelating agent, dithizone, which was dissolved in carbon tetrachloride (CCl_4). I would place the material in flasks with a drain apparatus at the bottom, shake them and place them upright and drain the carbon tetrachloride off. Then we would shake them again with dithizone and carbon tetrachloride. After three extractions theoretically we had removed all of the zinc from the water-soluble phase. The colored carbon tetrachloride was then read in quartz containers called cuvettes in a spectrophotometer at the peak wavelength of the zinc-dithizone complex and the concentration of zinc calculated from a calibration curve containing known amounts of zinc. It always concerned me that I was handling and breathing CCl_4 which is a toxin for the liver and kidneys.

I had to demonstrate that I was able to analyze ten zinc standards at one time to show that I could achieve 3 percent or less variation (repeatability). I then analyzed zinc standards on ten consecutive days to show that I could achieve 5 percent or less variation (reproducibility). Finally I measured the amount of zinc in a biological standard and achieved a result within 5 percent of the known value (accuracy). These terms in parenthesis are the foundation of methods in analytical chemistry. If we wanted to measure more than just zinc in a specimen then the material was ashed and analyzed in a large carbon-spark spectrograph which Dr. Vallee had developed and brought with him from MIT. This method developed on a long piece of film spectral band lines of all the different elements in the specimen. We learned to measure the density of the bands. This method allowed us to analyze multiple elements at one time. After a few months, I produced satisfactory analytical values for zinc.

Then Ralph Thiers and I began a new project in which I used radioactive ^{65}zinc hydroxide at a pH (acidity) where the zinc hydroxide was least soluble and formed a precipitate in a test tube. We measured the ^{65}zinc in the supernatant above the precipitate to calculate the solubility of zinc at the chosen pH of 8. When we mixed in a compound that bound zinc and shook the tube until the system came to equilibrium, we could calculate the binding constant or affinity of the compound for zinc by the amount of ^{65}zinc that appeared in the soluble supernatant above the zinc hydroxide precipitate. I spent three months trying to get binding constant values that coincided with published results without success. I finally found out that Dr. Thiers had given me the wrong pH to do the precipitation. I had not checked myself what the minimal solubility pH for zinc hydroxide was. My results were all erroneous. I learned an important lesson, which is never trust your adviser to tell you what the conditions of the experiment are when you are the one who is going to spend the time and effort doing the research.

Every Thursday night we had a laboratory meeting for all of the staff members and research fellows in the laboratory. Dr. Bert Vallee sat at a big table and ran the proceedings. He called on people without prior warning to present data on the work they were doing, including the plans of their experiment, the methods they were using, the results they had obtained and their interpretation of the results. It was understood that everything was up for question and discussion. I presented my results of the ^{65}zinc studies and everyone took turns criticizing what I was doing. I later found out that one of my fellow hospital residents had told Dr. Vallee privately that I was an assertive, bright, talkative "wise-guy" and that I would "take over the lab." No one could have said anything that would make Dr.

Vallee feel more negative about one of his laboratory fellows, because he was the absolute authority in our laboratory. This opinion about me filtered down to the other staff members of the laboratory and they were told to put me down and humble me whenever the opportunity came along. For some reason my personality and manner of speaking irritated Dr. Vallee. I decided that he wanted to break down what he perceived as my misplaced and false over-confidence and then build it back up again based on my success in the laboratory. The truth was that I was frightened of the people in the laboratory and in particular of Dr. Vallee. I was always doubtful of my ability to perform up to their standards.

Dr. Vallee closed the lab for the month of August and everyone went on vacation. I was then told that in the first year the fellows received no vacation but would have to wait until a year later. Therefore, everybody left and I was alone in the laboratory working all day and many evenings. Fortunately, my medical school classmate and internship buddy, Jim Adelstein, came by and helped counsel me. He had worked with Dr. Vallee when he was at MIT as an undergraduate and was now a senior resident. Believing that I would have August off, I had rented a cottage on Lake Sunapee in New Hampshire for the summer from the man who was the Chaplain at Kingsville Naval Air Station. Woody, Martha Sue and our new baby Jennifer went to the cottage and stayed there most of the summer. I would work Monday through Thursday day and night and then leave early Friday morning to drive to New Hampshire so that I could at least have the weekend with the family. Woody's father and stepmother came to visit us and a medical school classmate's wife also came with her children to spend a week. Unfortunately, the summer was cold and rainy.

In order to supplement my income, I took a job working in the Peter Bent Brigham Alcoholic Clinic on Tuesday nights between 6 and 9 p.m. We saw patients who were referred to the hospital because of uncontrolled alcohol abuse. We tried to help them by using psychotherapy and cognitive reality testing. We were supervised by an outstanding psychiatrist, David Myerson, who had been the state commissioner on alcohol problems and was a recognized expert in this disease. He taught me so much about alcoholic people, how to understand and help them and how to do reality testing when needed.

During that first year in the laboratory, I read many books on metal chemistry, on metalloenzymes and on analytical chemistry, and brushed up on my calculus. I worked one afternoon a week seeing patients in a liver clinic with Dr. Warren Wacker and this kept up my clinical skills. In the fall of 1957, I signed up as a special student at MIT and took one course per semester of advanced work for graduate students, such as an excellent course in enzymology and another on biophysical methods. During the fall, I was asked by someone among the resident group in the hospital to give them a talk on zinc deficiency and I was stupid enough to agree to do so. When Dr. Vallee heard about this, he angrily stopped my participation, pointing out that I was a beginner in the lab, that I had no great knowledge about zinc metabolism. He sent someone else in my place to give the talk.

All during the fall of 1957, I failed to find a project of my own which was productive. However, I continued to assay serum and urine zinc as part of a clinical study of zinc deficiency in alcoholic cirrhosis. I learned a great deal by listening to and hearing presentations about the experimental work of others. Every spring, the people in the laboratory worked hard to prepare talks which they would give at the American Society of Biological Chemists meetings in Atlantic City. I watched how the others learned to write these ten-minute talks, prepare their slides and deliver them in a way that the rest of the lab thought was acceptable. I unfortunately had no talk to give and went to Atlantic City feeling like one of the failures in the laboratory. Woody and I hosted a party for the lab in the Spring. Dr. Vallee asked her how I was adjusting to the lab. She pointed out that one of the things that made her fall in love with me was that I was always enthusiastic, cheerful and excited about medicine and biological problems. She said that ever since I had begun working in the laboratory, I was depressed and had lost my self-confidence. She wanted to know, "What are you doing to Phil?" Dr. Vallee was quite upset to hear this and I think he began to reconsider his pedagogical methods in my regard. Unfortunately, I would come home from the lab angry and depressed and my relationship with my wife and with my children deteriorated and after a while they could not stand to hear any more complaints about what was happening in my daily work in the lab.

Finally, in August of 1958, it came time for me to have a vacation. We rented a cottage in North Waterford, Maine, on the Five Kezar Ponds. The property was owned by a man named Bill Pettigrew who had built most of the cottages himself. His wife was a former teacher and a warm and motherly person. My children grew to love Bill and Lucy Pettigrew. I fished with my wife and children. We swam in the lake. We hiked on the hills and around the lake. It was probably the best vacation of my life. My sister Suzanne came to visit even though she was six months pregnant, and my parents visited us, and surprisingly we all got along well with one another and with the children. I felt refreshed and confident and when I went back to the laboratory I was determined to do a better job.

In September of 1958, I began a project making yeast alcohol dehydrogenase, an enzyme purified from yeast which we grew in the basement of the laboratory.

My partner in this effort was Dr. Jeremias H. R. Kaegi, a Swiss fellow from Zurich who became one of my best friends in the laboratory and subsequently. We would work all day and all night and the next day to get to the point in the preparation where we had crystals of the enzyme which were stable. We were successful in making high quality yeast alcohol dehydrogenase, which a number of people in the laboratory and I used for new research projects. I tried and failed to make alcohol dehydrogenase enzyme from a frozen beef liver which had been labeled with radioactive zinc. I used the method developed for horse liver. Unfortunately, in beef liver the activity was quite low compared to the horse liver, which has a remarkably high activity. I then began a project with a different staff member of the laboratory, Dr. Frederic L. Hoch, on the effects of silver and mercury on yeast alcohol dehydrogenase (YADH). It turned out that organic mercurials in particular would split the YADH into smaller subunits and this breakdown in the structure of the enzyme was reversible if chelating agents which removed the mercurials were added back quickly. I followed this change in structure by measuring the activity and the ultraviolet spectral changes. I found that the sulfhydryl (SH) amino acid glutathione reversed this loss of enzyme activity if it was added quickly enough to the mercurials or silver. This splitting of the protein was not reversed by adding zinc so it occurred at a different part of the enzyme than the zinc binding site. These mercurials or silver eventually led to a release of the firmly bound zinc, probably by pulling the protein apart. We studied the process in the ultracentrifuge where we were able to identify the breakdown of the normal size YADH into smaller species secondary to the loss of zinc. All of this work preceded later knowledge that YADH was a polymer of four similar subunits held together in part by sulfur-sulfur bonds which are disrupted by mercurials. Dr. Hoch and I wrote up this work and presented it in a talk in Atlantic City which was published in the Federation Proceedings of 1959. I was standing in a large auditorium with many prominent biochemists sitting in the front row who asked me many difficult questions about the work. I was so frightened that a picture that Dr. Hoch took showed that the color of my face was as white as that of the projection screen. However, I held my own answering the questions and the people from the laboratory congratulated me on doing a good piece of work. This paper which we wrote on this research was accepted for publication in the *Journal of Biological Chemistry* in August of 1959 and finally published in February of 1960. This research and publication was essentially my only success from two years in the laboratory.

During the year that I was a junior resident and the first year in the lab while I was doing everything else, I collected at night from hospital records the clinical findings of 400 patients who had serum lactic dehydrogenase (LDH) assays performed in the laboratory. These patients had a broad spectrum of diseases. After Drs. Vallee and Wacker looked at all the data that I had accumulated we decided that the best use of the LDH assay was in the diagnosis of an acute heart attack or myocardial infarction, where we had proof of the diagnosis in 34 patients. After ten drafts of the paper, each one rejected in turn by Dr. Vallee, he finally allowed me to send it to the *New England Journal of Medicine*, where it was accepted and published in December of 1959. It showed that the serum LDH assay was a sensitive but not specific detector of myocardial infarction, similar to but more sensitive than the serum glutamic oxalacetic transaminase assay that others had used. Soon the LDH assay was used throughout the country. Unfortunately it was also elevated in many other illnesses. Serum enzyme assays more specific for the heart muscle were eventually developed.

Looking back on my two years in the Biophysics Laboratory, I believe that I learned how to do good research, to run a laboratory, to direct technicians in their work and how to plan, carry out, present and publish results of research. I was not productive myself but I see that to some extent this was due to poor choice of projects by Dr. Vallee and by myself. Unfortunately I never won his or the other staff people's respect as far as my research was concerned. I felt like a failure compared to the other fellows who had gone through the lab or were going through the lab with me. I seriously questioned whether I should do laboratory research in biochemistry as part of my future career. I did make close friends among a few of the lab members, in particular Warren Wacker, who had worked with me before as a resident, Jerry Kaegi and Jim Adelstein. I never did learn to relate constructively to my boss, Dr. Bert L. Vallee. I think there was an intrinsic conflict between our personalities. However, he supported my nomination to be chief medical resident later and to be appointed Chief of Gastroenterology after that. He showed loyalty to his former fellows, even those like me who did not do well in the laboratory years. I accepted a senior resident position for the year 1959–1960 rather than spending another year in the Biophysics Research Laboratory and this clinical year began on July 1, 1959.

7

Senior Residency

✦

1959–1960

I was assigned to the West Roxbury Veterans Administration (VA) Hospital for the first four months of 1959. The day I took over the ward from the previous senior resident, Dr. David Nathan, he told me that he tried to clear out the ward of patients who were ready to go home or shouldn't have been in the ward in the first place. He sent 16 patients home the day that I arrived and by evening, the people in the admitting room had admitted 16 more patients to fill up the beds. Many of the people who came in did not need to be in the hospital but the rule was to keep all beds full or the hospital would not get full funding from the VA. My junior residents were Thorne Winter and William Hood, who had both interned at the Brigham. As medical students they had taken part in the experimental program in Bert Vallee's lab whereby medical students were taught third-year internal medicine integrated with basic science. They were both conscientious and bright people and we had a wonderful time together. I thought the West Roxbury VA hospital was somewhat better than it was in 1956 and 1957. We now could get clinical chemistry results performed in the hospital on nights and weekends and emergency services were better for X-ray and other laboratory tests.

I began to share rides to the hospital from Belmont with Dr. David Littmann, who was the Chief of Cardiology at the West Roxbury. He pioneered cardiac catheterization and coronary angiography at the VA hospital and in Boston. He also invented a lightweight and efficient stethoscope that is now used widely in the United States and throughout the world. Dave had coronary artery disease himself but he acted as his own physician and took no treatment other than nitroglycerin tablets. We would drive through Watertown Square in the morning rush-hour traffic in his sports car when he would become angry with the other drivers who were cutting in on him. Then he developed chest pain. He did not stop but popped a nitroglycerin under his tongue and kept on driving. I became quite concerned about his health, but he would not take my advice and find a good personal cardiologist.

He conducted famous teaching conferences on electrocardiography for the junior and senior residents. I still remembered many of his most difficult tracings from my junior residency rotation. When the residents had made their guesses at the correct reading, he would call on me and I would give the correct answer. We laughed together about this because I was known as an ordinary electrocardiographer. Dave Littmann lived for a number of years more before he died of a heart attack (myocardial infarction).

My relationship with the Chief of the Medical Service, Dr. Thomas Warthin, was no better than it was when I was a junior resident. He took great pride that he was an oral examiner for the Board of Internal Medicine and showed me his collection of unusual X-rays that he showed to candidates. I remember that one was an X-ray of the spine with calcified intervertebral discs due to ochronosis, a rare genetic defect also called alcaptonuria. He seemed pleased that he could fail so many candidates with his unusual cases. A few years later the Board gave up oral exams because of unfair examiners like Dr. Warthin. He did a good share of general internal medicine attending on our wards. Unfortunately he was becoming out of date and often gave us incorrect information.

Ira Gore was the Chief of Pathology and a collector of rare diseases. He wrote a paper on a condition called atheromatous embolization due to atherosclerotic aortic plaques that showered pieces of cholesterol into various organs, especially the kidneys and pancreas, and into the lower legs and feet. This condition was rarely diagnosed during life. I cared for an old man on the ward with fat and undigested meat fibers in his feces who we proved had pancreatic insufficiency, as well as mild kidney failure. We could find no other reasons for these problems. I postulated and Dr. Gore agreed that he might have the atheromatous embolization syndrome. A subsequent autopsy showed atrophy of the pancreas due to many cholesterol emboli blocking the blood vessels. He also had renal failure due to these cholesterol emboli. We learned a good deal of standard pathology from Dr. Gore's autopsy conferences, although he showed so many slides of the same findings that many of us fell asleep during the conferences. Still, the VA was a storehouse of unusual pathologic material.

A merchant marine seaman was admitted to the hospital with a pox-like rash over his body and somebody feared that this might be smallpox (variola major). We put him on very strict isolation and called Dr. Louis Weinstein, our infectious disease consultant who pointed out that the lesions were occurring in one crop after another and were particularly dense on the trunk and that there were early papules before poxes developed. He made the correct diagnosis of chicken pox (varicella) which was disseminated in this adult who may have been immunocompromised. All of us were relieved since most of us had already had chicken pox. I thought my four-month experience at the VA was quite valuable because we had a chance to do long-term observation and management of diseases. Some of the patients I kept the entire four months that I was there until their problems were resolved. Most veteran patients were grateful for the care that they received and cooperative with their doctors. The main drawback was dealing with the VA bureaucracy, which had not improved since 1956.

In November of 1959, I returned to the Brigham and was assigned to E-Main, the main female ward. There I found the same population of 70- to 90-year-old women, many from nursing homes, that I had encountered when I was an intern. These elderly women were sent in with various infections, strokes, heart attacks, heart failure and cancers and we struggled to prolong their sometimes miserable lives. My interns were Ting Kai Li (known as T.K.) and Bernard Babior, two of the brightest people in one of the best intern groups I can recall at the Brigham. Besides T.K. Li and Bernie Babior, they included Robert Blacklow, Joseph Pines, Joseph Pittman, Charles Epstein, James Ryan, Lincoln Potter, Fred Welland, and Norman Lasser. Ting Kai had come to the Biophysics Research Laboratory as a second year Harvard medical student for an experimental program where Dr. Vallee and Dr. Warren Wacker taught physical diagnosis in the second year and general internal medicine in the third year to a group of four students. They combined the teaching of clinical subjects with a heavy dose of basic science linked to clinical medicine. It seemed to work quite successfully for those people who went through this program. I knew T.K. because of his outstanding student research project in the Biophysics lab on liver alcohol dehydrogenase. As my intern he became and has remained these many years one of my good friends and a colleague in science whom I turned to when I needed thoughtful and critical advice.

Bernie Babior was a tough, smart graduate of UCLA and he and I had our disagreements. Once he purposefully neglected to call me about an admission of a woman to E-Main so that I could examine her. I was left to explain who this person might be at morning report. Back on the ward I lost my temper and chewed him out for his lack of cooperation. He said that he didn't need my help and that he could work up these patients without calling me. I suggested that we go outside behind the ward and have it out with our fists if he would not play by the rules. With this threat he backed down and we finally worked out a testy relationship. Bernie Babior finished his residency at the Boston City Hospital and then went on to get basic science training that eventually led him to become Chief of Molecular and Experimental Medicine at Scripps Research Institute in La Jolla, California.

During the second month Robert Blacklow joined us as Babior left. I knew Bob from his time in medical school. He was very bright. He was a close friend of T.K. Li. They were quite a pair and gave me a run for my money. The patient who stands out during those two months was one admitted to T.K., a 21-year-old girl with systemic lupus erythematosus and lupus nephritis, in early renal failure. T.K. put her on high doses of corticosteroids and finally got her into remission. She went home but unfortunately relapsed and later died of complications of lupus, especially the renal failure. T.K. proved to be a caring and thoughtful physician, wise beyond his years.

The ward on E-Main always contained a group of elderly Jewish ladies, usually with heart disease, who argued frequently about who was of higher social status when they lived back in Kiev in Russia. Stanley James Adelstein, my classmate and friend from the Biophysics lab, was our chief resident. In 1957 he married a wonderful woman named Mary Taylor, an editor at one of the publishing houses in Boston. Jim was given only one weekend off for his honeymoon and a fellow resident covered for him the Friday of the wedding. The other senior residents were Martin Liebowitz, my former intern; Phil Bromberg, my classmate at Harvard and fellow intern in 1953–54, who had been doing pulmonary research with Dr. Burwell and Eugene Robin; John Downey from Manitoba, who worked with me at the West Roxbury for four months and later went on to become Professor of Rehabilitation Medicine at Columbia Physicians and Surgeons medical school; James E. C. Walker from the University of Pennsylvania, Wisconsin, and Michigan, who later became Professor at the University of Connecticut School of Medicine; and Sidney Wanzer, who trained at the Brigham and after finishing his senior residency actually practiced internal medicine in Concord, Massachusetts, and worked part-time at the Harvard Health Services, both at the college and at the law school.

Jim Adelstein initiated monthly dinners held at Jim Walker's beautiful apartment in the Back Bay wherein we senior residents invited senior faculty to dine and talk with us. Our guests included George Packer Berry, dean of Harvard Medical School; George W. Thorn, who bankrolled these soirees; and Francis D. Moore and Samuel A. Levine. They all seemed to enjoy the dinners, wine, cigars, brandy and conversation as much as we did. The wives of the senior residents were asked to prepare the dinners! My wife questioned this arrangement, considering it an imposition on working women or women with children when they were not invited to join the dinners.

After E-Main, I moved to the private service during January and February of 1960, where I was on call every other night and weekend admitting patients to either E-Main or F-Main. One evening Richard Russell, a junior resident, and I saw a surgical intern taking a student nurse up to his room in the doctors' quarters. Rich told me that they had a saying in Alabama where he came from that "You should never get your honey where you make your money." I passed this wisdom on to my students and residents.

On January 18th, my third daughter was born at the Boston Lying-In Hospital by natural childbirth, something rarely seen there because the deliveries were almost always with the mother under deep anesthesia, having been premedicated with scopolamine and Demerol. The babies ordinarily were sluggish and rather blue when they came out and required a good deal of stimulation to get them to breathe. Dr. Brian Little agreed to deliver the baby by natural childbirth at my wife's request. He invited the medical students and nursing students to observe her delivery because it was so unusual. The baby came out pink and looked all around at the lights and hardly cried at all. After Dr. Little announced that we had a third daughter, he asked, "What is her name?" When my wife said that we are going to call her Amy, he picked her up and danced around the room to show her to everybody, singing "Once in Love with Amy."

I missed this marvelous experience because I had admitted a patient to T.K. Li, an 18-year-old single Italian girl who had tried to perform an abortion on herself with a coat hanger. She perforated her uterus and developed an abscess and sepsis due to *Clostridium perfringens*, the organism that causes gas gangrene. The infection also included a streptoccocal organism. We could not convince the Chief of Obstetrics at the Boston Lying-In, Dr. Duncan Reid, to do an emergency hysterectomy because he said she was too unstable. So all night we dealt with her low blood pressure (septic shock). We gave her fluids and high doses of penicillin and other broad-spectrum antibiotics. By dint of prolonged good care, she eventually recovered. They called me from the Boston Lying-In at four in the morning to tell me that I had a third daughter when I was hoping for a son. I said "damn" and hung up. After I got to the hospital the next morning and saw Amy, such a beautiful baby girl, I apologized to my wife and to Dr. Little and welcomed this third offspring into our family.

While on the private service, no problems arose between me and certain private doctors. I learned to correct their mistakes and to point them out to no one. In May and June I was back on F-Main, where I had started at the Brigham as an intern. This time, my interns were Joseph Pines and Joseph Pittman, two very bright and assertive interns who now felt that they knew enough to run the ward without me. We had arguments on work rounds because I verbally checked on what they were doing. I found that being a publicly compulsive resident only engendered resentment and an unpleasant atmosphere on the ward. I stopped checking on them openly, instead looking quietly into the hospital records and the orders that they wrote. Joe Pines became a cardiologist who practiced at Beth Israel Hospital in the Harvard system and Joe Pittman became an endocrinologist and later dean of the branch of the Illinois Medical School in Rockford, Illinois. Charles Epstein, one of the other outstanding interns, later became a victim of a terrorist called the Unabomber, whose actual name was Ted Kaczynski. He randomly chose Dr. Epstein, by then a prominent geneticist, to receive a bomb in a package. When Charlie opened the package, the explosion caused him severe hand and facial injuries, but he continued to work as Professor of Pediatrics and as a geneticist at the University of California in San Francisco. Unfortunately I never knew what became of the other interns in this class.

In the last week of my residency, I was hospitalized with a resistant *Staphylococcus aureus* infection on my arm and was treated with broad-spectrum antibiotics. After I left on vacation I developed prolonged and severe diarrhea. We would now know that this was due to antibiotic-induced *Clostridium difficile* overgrowth and release of its toxin in the colon.

In 1960 in July when I returned from vacation, I began a one-year fellowship to work with Warren Wacker in his own laboratory across from Dr. Burwell's laboratory. I was given a Russell Stearns Fellowship to support me during that year. I worked with Elias Amador, a pathologist, and with a Dr. John Peterson, who was chairman of medicine at Loma Linda Medical School in Los Angeles. John was on sabbatical, working with Warren. Elias, John and I became longtime good friends. I measured zinc in the serum and urine of patients with alcoholic cirrhosis, whom we treated with oral zinc. I confirmed the increased urinary zinc excretion in the urine in spite of a low serum zinc which Drs. Vallee and Wacker had reported in alcoholic cirrhosis. Unexpectedly I found it occurred in other forms of cirrhosis. There was some lessening of the zinc in the urine as the patients stopped drinking and took oral zinc but it was not clear that the oral zinc was therapeutic.

During that year I helped Warren Wacker publish in the *Journal of the American Medical Association* a series of patients who had pulmonary embolism or pulmonary infarction, gleaned from the four hundred cases that I had reviewed who had serum LDH measurements made in the Biophysics laboratory from 1956 to

1959. We had six autopsy-proven cases and eleven highly probable clinical cases and all showed elevated serum LDH levels. However, this also occurred in acute myocardial infarctions so we needed a way to separate the two. We noted that in our patients and in the reports in the literature there was often a rise in serum bilirubin, usually below jaundice levels in patients with pulmonary infarction, and no rise in the serum glutamic oxalacetic transaminase (SGOT), an enzyme activity that is elevated in heart attacks. We proposed a diagnostic triad for pulmonary infarction, namely an elevated serum LDH, elevated serum bilirubin and a normal SGOT. This publication aroused interest and controversy throughout the U.S. I was asked to give a talk on our research at Massachusetts General at their grand rounds in the Ether Dome, a singular honor.

During that year, I found that patients with hemochromatosis, the iron storage disease, had a deficiency of zinc in their livers, a low serum zinc and increased zinc in their urine. I thought that this was due to iron competition against zinc storage in liver but I never published this information. I was also given the job of supervising the Brigham clinical chemistry laboratory. I found myself interceding between the lab technicians and the interns and residents, who differed about what tests were emergencies and which results they believed were valid. I studied to improve my knowledge of analytical chemistry so that I could improve the methods that we were using and define statistically the normal values for our laboratory. The chief technician was a competent and intelligent woman trained in Denmark named Kirsten Hviid. She and I published a paper together in the *Journal of Laboratory and Clinical Medicine* in 1962 which showed that the new automated flame photometer, which had just come on the market, gave valid measures for sodium and potassium compared to the old manual flame photometer or our laboratory flame spectrometer. During this year George Thorn offered me the Chief Residency for 1961–1962 and I happily accepted.

During the wait to begin my Chief Residency I reviewed three years of autopsy reports, looking for medical problems that could be treated more successfully. The two that I chose were pulmonary embolism and bacterial sepsis caused by Gram-negative organisms. A high degree of suspicion and aggressive diagnostic and therapeutic methods were reported to reduce mortality in pulmonary embolism. Early diagnosis and aggressive treatment of Gram-negative sepsis with kanamycin and its later antibiotic descendants were able to save many of these patients, although this class of antibiotics could cause severe kidney and hearing damage. I planned to devote my residency to attacking these two clinical problems that our autopsy files showed we were managing poorly.

8

Chief Residency

◆

1961–1963

An appointment as Chief Resident in Medicine was considered a great honor at the Peter Bent Brigham Hospital. Dr. George Thorn chose his chief residents with the advice of his Department of Medicine senior professors. Dr. Bert Vallee told me that Dr. Thomas Warthin from the West Roxbury VA hospital spoke against me in the conference and that cinched my candidacy because Dr. Warthin was so unpopular with the other senior physicians. Why did Dr. Thorn choose me? I was always respectful toward him but I never curried favor as did some other residents. I think that Bert Vallee and Warren Wacker recommended me and that carried a good deal of weight. For reasons that I will never understand, George Thorn liked and trusted me. Dr. Eugene Eppinger, who had been a chief resident in the 1930s, also supported me and advised me that the job was "the care and feeding of the interns and residents."

My intern class of twelve consisted of John Milner, John Moxley, Shaun Ruddy, Richard Tannen, John Wilber, James Mertz, Richard Lewis, Robert Young, Ralph Himmelhoch, Arthur Gottlieb, Martin Cohen and Arthur Baker. At the Brigham the key people needed for a chief resident to succeed were the senior residents. My excellent group of six were Thomas O'Brien, Hugh McDevitt, Guillermo (Bill) Herrera, William (Bucky) Greenough, Victor Sidel and Paul Jagger. The junior resident group had grown to fourteen in number as we opened new rotations and the Brigham affiliated with more hospitals. During the first week, I lived in the chief resident's quarters on the third floor of the house staff dormitory area and roamed the wards day and night to see how the new people were doing.

The chief resident chose the cases or topics for the Friday medical grand rounds held in the main amphitheater between 10:30 a.m. and noon, and also scheduled the speakers. We usually had two case presentations or subjects and two speakers. Surgical grand rounds moved to Saturday mornings, giving us the luxury of 1.5 hours for medical grand rounds. In the summer I scheduled sessions on basic science which related to medicine and asked professors from the medical school to talk, one of them being my friend Harold Amos from bacteriology, who talked about the exciting new topic of viral phage infections. The list of speakers in 1961–1962 was amazing. I could convince almost anyone in Boston to discuss patients whose diseases were among their favorite topics.

On Wednesday noon we presented medical pathological conferences, usually accompanied by the autopsy or surgical findings of a deceased patient. The topics covered every area of medicine and neurology and some surgery. I was able to recruit discussers from the entire Boston medical community and visiting professors from the U.S. and abroad as well as the Brigham staff. I also used this conference to have the residents discuss their own cases and sometimes I was the discusser. On Wednesday afternoons the medical house staff and pathologists assembled in the Pathology department to view the gross and microscopic findings on our autopsied patients. By discussing any errors in clinical management in privacy, we were able to share our outcomes with one another and learn from each other.

On Thursday afternoons at Dr. Thorn's suggestion we presented "Medical Teas," in which three interns, residents, fellows, staff or visitors made fifteen-minute presentations on research topics followed by discussion, both in basic and clinical science. The expertise among our house staff and fellows was amazing.

The chief resident was also responsible for choosing the cases and writing up the case summaries for the clinical pathological conferences (CPCs) held every two weeks at noon on Mondays. I had filed away my dictated discharge summaries since my internship and used many of these for CPCs. I sometimes asked staff members to discuss patients whom they had seen in consultation or ones who were their own private patients but whose outcome they did not know because they were absent from the hospital when they died. One of these cases was an elderly woman admitted to the private service by our infectious disease specialist, who was her family doctor. She spent a month on the ward gradually becoming more and more ill from some kind of pneumonia, which was unresponsive to our usual antibiotics. Her doctor went on vacation and when she died the autopsy showed that she had pulmonary tuberculosis in a rare lobar pneumonia form. Many interns, residents, and nurses became infected while caring for her and their tuberculin tests turned positive. As chief resident it was my responsibility to treat them for a year with isoniazid and para-aminosalicylic acid because of the new positive tuberculin tests or a new lung lesion on chest X-rays. When I asked the infectious disease doctor to discuss this case, he again missed the diagnosis!

One of the aggravating problems about grand rounds was when a person scheduled to be one of the two speakers canceled at the last minute. To cover this problem, I had certain staff members who liked to talk at grand rounds and had "cookbook" talks on subjects in their specialty ready to go. They usually agreed to discuss a case or topic on short notice, but their talks were often ones we had heard before. Once when all else failed, I gave a discussion of a case of Thorazine-induced liver injury, which I had researched in a few days.

Each morning, I came to F-main and E-main, the large public wards, and briefly talked with and examined the new patients who were admitted during the past 24 hours. Then I went to morning report with the senior residents, who presented their cases to Dr. Thorn or the acting chief of medicine. I prided myself on occasionally recognizing a disease not considered by my house staff. One example which impressed my F-main team was a man with headaches and confusion. I detected that he had paralysis of conjugate upward gaze; in other words, he could not look upward with both eyes together. I wrote a short note suggesting that he must have a brain tumor in the pineal region, which turned out to be the case. Most of my quick pickups were due to asking the right questions or looking for the physical signs I thought should be present. It became a contest to prevent me from out-guessing my interns and residents so they made even greater efforts in their workups.

We had house staff meetings every week where problems and issues were discussed. Some issues involved our fourth-year Harvard Medical School students who were assigned as clinical clerks to teams on F-main and E-main. One young woman student repeatedly was absent from the ward and her duties. She explained to me that she had contracted infectious mononucleosis six months ago and had never recovered her energy or her ability to concentrate. I looked up her record at the medical school health service. She had never had a proven diagnosis of infectious mononucleosis with a typical history, physical examination and a positive heterophile antibody. She had missed time in all her courses since the illness, yet all her laboratory tests were normal. I graded the fourth-year students for Dr. Thorn and gave her an incomplete, meaning that she would have to repeat the two months of fourth-year medicine. She was very angry and went to the medical school student dean, who called me over to defend my grade. She accused me of being prejudiced against female students. The dean asked me to pass her as the other course directors had been doing for the past six months. I refused and Dr. Thorn backed me up. I now suspect that she had chronic fatigue syndrome, a mysterious disabling set of symptoms, sometimes erroneously called chronic infectious mononucleosis. This syndrome is of unknown cause and no treatment was available then or now for this condition. I do not recall if she graduated from Harvard Medical School or had to repeat some of her other courses. Objectively, she did not meet the acceptable performance of a clinical clerk on medicine. These problems with certain students caused me great anguish because I had been in their position a few years earlier. I met weekly with the students to discuss their patients and have them present a talk about the clinical picture, diagnosis and treatment of their patients' problems. I learned to know them fairly well and many of them became my friends and eventually members of the Brigham house staff.

Ralph Himmelhoch, one of my interns, and a surgical resident designed and carried out a prospective trial of the new procedure called cardiopulmonary resuscitation (CPR). They alternated night duties so one could be present at every cardiac arrest and carry out their protocol properly. They standardized cardiac compression, direct current defibrillation and drug therapy. After six months and about a hundred patients they analyzed their results and published them in the *New England Journal of Medicine.* They found that aged patients and those with cancer, pneumonia or heart failure rarely left the hospital after CPR. The appropriateness of CPR in certain patients became an ethical issue and led to the development of "do not resuscitate" orders. This is a prime example of Dr. Thorn's policy of encouragement of clinical research by house staff.

Dr. Thorn heard through the grapevine at the National Institutes of Health that the Clinical Centers branch was about to fund clinical research centers outside the NIH campus and that Johns Hopkins hospital was to receive the first one. Applications for such centers were open to other hospitals but the opportunity was barely advertised and the deadline was within a few days. At Dr. Thorn's request Bert Vallee, Warren Wacker and Jim Adelstein met in his office on Friday, Saturday and Sunday and worked nonstop to write an application for a 24-bed research ward at the Brigham, listing many novel kinds of projects not done in clinical research anywhere else. The huge application was typed and then mailed from the Boston airport at midnight Sunday to meet the Monday deadline. I heard that the people at NIH were astounded to receive this unsolicited application. It was approved by the review committee, funding with millions of dollars the entire 24-bed ward along with supporting laboratories. The main female ward, E-Main, was taken to create this 24-bed Clinical Center, and E-2 and F-2 semiprivate wards were converted to public female wards. The basement of E-Main was converted into the supporting laboratories. At that time the Brigham was near bankruptcy and the NIH grant helped solve the financial crisis.

During 1962–1963, Dr. Thorn decided to take a sabbatical year to travel and study, and to become a guest member in the Biophysics Research Laboratory. When he was in town, he attended the Thursday evening lab meetings and worked with certain staff members as an adviser on their projects. His presence put a damper on Dr. Vallee's assertive criticism of people's work. He asked me to stay on for a second year of chief residency, stating that he did not want a new chief resident to face the year without his support and presence. He asked Dr. Eugene Eppinger to be the acting chief of the Department of Medicine.

My new intern class of thirteen was outstanding. The Harvard Medical School grads were Andrew Kang, Robert Dluhy, Kenneth McIntosh, Morton Goldberg and Burton Sobel. The others were Michael Herman, Jay Sullivan, Charles Blair, Richard Carruthers, Warren Davis, James Dodge, Matthew Menken and Scott Murphy. My senior residents were known to me from the time they had spent as interns, junior residents or specialty fellows. They were Sidney Alexander, William Hood, Robert Druyan, Earle Hammer, Leon Sabath and Charles Hollander.

The second year went more smoothly than the first because I had learned how to lead and be supportive and still allow people to grow on their own. However, one of my interns struggled to keep up with the workload. A fellow intern asked me to come to his room in the dormitory in September. There was his bed, carefully made up and not slept in. The window was open and a bird had made a nest on his pillow. The other intern thought that this man always stayed up all night when on duty. Dr. Samuel Bojar, who had been trained as an internist and then become a psychiatrist, was our house staff psychiatric advisor. I arranged for him to talk with this troubled intern, who told him that all the other interns were smarter than he was and even if he worked day and night he could never equal the performance of the others. He never felt he was in control of his patient load. By this time, he was quite depressed. Dr. Bojar and I reassured him that he was doing a good job of patient care by all reports. He said that he did not plan to accept a junior residency but wanted to join the U.S. Army Medical Corps the next year, where he felt he could excel. I was still concerned about his depression and put a suicide watch on him. I asked the interns and residents rotating with him to check on him frequently and make sure that he was rarely alone. The reason I was so concerned is that in 1954 a graduate from Harvard Medical School named Kenneth Borg, who had been at Kirkland house with me at Harvard College, came to the Brigham as an intern. He became depressed and in August leaped from the window of his third-floor house staff room, impaling himself on the spikes of the iron fence below. This horrible story haunted me and made me determined to avoid another suicide. Our troubled intern began to enjoy his work, finished out the year and joined the Army Medical Corps. I heard that he became a full colonel and was a great success in that structured environment.

Early in the year, Morton Goldberg told me about a 50-year-old woman in his outpatient clinic who he found had an elevated serum calcium level. He looked for a parathyroid tumor and none was apparent. Because of red cells in the urine, he obtained an intravenous pyelogram and found a mass in the kidney, presumably a kidney cancer. He suspected that the tumor might be the cause of her high serum calcium because tumors of other organs produced hormones, so-called para-neoplastic hormone production. He asked if I knew anyone in Boston who could assay parathyroid hormone and fortunately I knew Armen H. Tashjian, Jr., who was a professor at Harvard Dental School. He had developed a bioassay for parathyroid-like hormones. The patient went to surgery, the tumor was removed and part was given to Dr. Tashjian for extraction of parathyroid-like hormones and for his bioassay. The tumor was read by the pathologist as a garden-variety renal cell cancer. Morton Goldberg and Armen Tashjian decided to publish this case when the parathyroid assay returned positive because it would be the first tumor producing a parathyroid-like hormone outside of the parathyroid glands. I got a call from the chairman of pathology, Gustave Dammin, who heard that the case was going to be published. He asked that Morton Goldberg include as coauthors his pathologist who read the slides and himself as Chief of Pathology. Next I got a call from Dr. Francis Moore, Chief of Surgery, who said he wanted the urological surgeon who removed the tumor and himself to be coauthors because the surgery was done on his service. Then Dr. Thorn called me because he had heard rumors about this case. I told him the story and he said that if all these other people were going to be coauthors he wanted the Department of Medicine to be represented by a senior person, namely himself, as senior author. The paper was published in the *American Journal of Medicine* a year later as the first case of parathyroid hormone-like material from a non-parathyroid tumor. The first author was Mort Goldberg, who actually wrote the paper. The second author was Armen Tashjian, followed by the pathologists, surgeons, and last George Thorn. This was a great lesson for Mort Goldberg and me about how academic doctors may try to climb aboard every time there is an important paper to be published. Mort went on to an ophthalmology residency at Johns Hopkins Hospital in the Wilmer Eye Institute, as he had planned, and rose to be chief resident there. After a distinguished career in clinical and research ophthalmology, he was called back to Johns Hopkins to be chairman of the Ophthalmology department at the Wilmer institute.

In 1999, I developed macular degeneration in my right eye and called my colleague from the Navy, John Eisenlohr, a former chief resident at the Wilmer, for advice about where to go for treatment. He referred me to a Dr. Goldberg, chief at the Wilmer, whose department had pioneered in the new treatment with photodynamic therapy. Dr. Goldberg said on the telephone, "Is this my old chief resident, Phil Snodgrass?" I said "Is this Mort Goldberg, my old intern?" When he saw me in his clinic, we laughed about the saga of his first paper and I told the story to his residents as a lesson in the aggressive way academic doctors try to get a free ride on others' important publications. Mort then told us a story about Dr. Samuel Levine. He called Dr. Levine when he was an intern because one of his inpatients had a slightly low serum potassium level. Dr. Levine told Mort "give him two bananas and call me in the morning" (bananas are rich in potassium). Incidentally, Dr. Goldberg's skillful photodynamic treatments stabilized the vision in my right eye.

I was asked to sit in on the interviews of students for their internships in the month of December. The system was then like the one I went through, with six teams of interviewers, a private meeting with Dr. Thorn and a meeting afterward to rate the students from 1 to 50. Only the top thirty had a chance of being one of our ten interns because our positions were highly sought after. One of our fourth-year students, named Marshall Wolf, was a Harvard Medical School graduate and a summa cum laude in chemistry from Harvard College. His senior chemistry professor at the college had written that he would not be a good doctor because he lacked empathy and should become a PhD chemist. I knew Marshall well and argued strongly that he had empathy, skill, and sensitivity, and was already showing the signs of being a good physician. He was finally passed by the group and given the low number (high rating) he deserved. Marshall interned in 1963–64, finished his residencies and cardiology fellowships at the Brigham, practiced cardiology there, became the associate chief of the Department of Medicine at the Brigham and for many years was its beloved house staff coordinator.

The chief resident was sometimes called upon to substitute for staff physicians who were unavailable and this finally happened to me. A 35-year-old man was admitted on a Saturday with recurrent ventricular tachycardia, a heart rhythm disturbance which had been continuing for many days at a rate of 200 beats per minute. The man was in mild heart failure. Ventricular tachycardia is dangerous because it can degenerate into ventricular fibrillation, a fatal rhythm disturbance. The cardiologist to whom he was referred, Dr. Harold Levine, was not in the hospital. When I reached Dr. Levine by phone, he asked me to go ahead and use the newly developed direct current defibrillator to shock the man out of this abnormal rhythm. It took three shocks with three hundred watt seconds, the full power setting, to induce him back into normal (sinus) heart rhythm. I was somewhat angry but also flattered to be asked to do this procedure when I was not an experienced cardiologist. We then began a drug called quinidine, the only one then available that might prevent him from having further bouts of ventricular tachycardia.

One morning as I walked down the basement corridor under the wards, I heard a call for help from the technician in the Allergy Laboratory. She had given a dose of pollen extract to a student nurse that by mistake was 100 times stronger than that intended. The nurse collapsed in the corridor in anaphylactic shock. I reached her first, began cardiopulmonary resuscitation and asked the technician to fill a syringe with one ml. of 1:1000 epinephrine. George Cahill, my former intern buddy, joined me and was able to get an intravenous infusion of saline going. He gave her the epinephrine through the tubing and then ordered and gave her 100 mg of hydrocortisone. In a few minutes she regained a good blood pressure and began to breathe normally. We took her to the emergency ward and with more epinephrine and an antihistamine she recovered completely. It was good fortune that George and I happened to be in the corridor at that time and at that place.

In November, one of my junior residents, Richard Tannen, came to see me and explained that he had just begun a new rotation at the Robert Breck Brigham Hospital, our affiliate which specialized in joint diseases like rheumatoid arthritis. When he went to examine the patients who were turned over to him by the previous resident, three patients asked him, "Why are you looking in my eyes? Why are you doing a rectal exam? Why are you listening to my heart?" The previous resident had not done these procedures, according to these patients. When Dick Tannen looked at the dictated and typed admission workups of this previous resident they clearly stated "fundal exam negative, rectal exam negative, heart exam negative." When Dick looked at previous hospital admission summaries, this junior resident's dictations were almost word for word similar to those on the old admissions. He brought me copies of the workups of the preceding resident and those done during previous admissions. I took this story and the evidence to Dr. Eugene Eppinger, who was acting chief of medicine while Dr. Thorn was on sabbatical. He asked me what we should do. I recommended discharging this resident who had faked his workups. We interviewed him and he explained that these patients were admitted every few months so in his opinion a complete physical examination was not necessary and he simply re-dictated the previous examination. It was a rule of our medicine training program that every new admission must have a new history and physical exam performed and entered in the medical record. I had known this man as a medical student and as a student researcher in Bert Vallee's laboratory. There he was caught making up results and almost burned up the cold room by his carelessness. He accused me of being against him on these grounds. Dr. Eppinger refused to fire him, but called Dr. Thorn in Arizona, where he was lecturing. He told Dr. Eppinger not to fire the resident but leave it to me to deal with the situation. After considerable thought, I removed him from the remaining rotations where he would care for patients and arranged for him to spend the next six months in pathology, where as I told him he could not kill anyone by his unprofessional behavior. The other residents were angry with me because they had to cover his rotations and give up their special electives that they had arranged. The resident in trouble finished the year in pathology and left the Brigham for his senior residency at another hospital. Subsequently, he specialized in pharmacology and eventually became chairman of pharmacology in a large state medical school. He has hated me ever since this sad incident. I only hoped that he learned from it and would cut no more corners during his further career.

In February, Robert Frost, the famous American poet, was admitted to A-Third with prostate cancer. He had complained of bouts of shortness of breath and vague chest pains. He was cared for by a committee of a urological surgeon, a cardiologist, an endocrinologist and an internist. I talked to him and reviewed his chart and became convinced that he was having multiple pulmonary emboli. I asked Warren Wacker to review the data and he agreed. He talked to Dr. Thorn about our concerns and pointed out that he had the elevated serum LDH and bilirubin and normal SGOT we had described as well as other clues by history, EKG and chest X-ray. The physician team caring for him never agreed with our diagnosis. When he died the autopsy showed multiple pulmonary emboli. This taught me that too many physicians, like too many cooks, can "spoil the broth."

During this year, I selected and wrote the case summaries for our clinical pathological conferences (CPCs). Surprisingly, I was able to convince Dr. Thorn to discuss a case. He had assiduously avoided this exercise in the past. I found a female patient with a slowly progressive history of seizures, confusion and dementia, renal failure, low platelet counts and occasional red spots on her lower legs. This was due to a rare disease called chronic thrombotic thrombocytopenic purpura (TTP). When Dr. Thorn began his discussion by saying, "The important point of these CPCs is not the correct diagnosis but the correct approach to the patient," I knew that he did not have a clue to the diagnosis in this case. I asked if any of the fourth-year clinical clerks taking medicine at the Brigham had submitted their diagnoses for this CPC. To my dismay, one of them called it chronic TTP. The autopsy findings showed the typical hyaline thrombi in small vessels of TTP due to platelet agglutination throughout the body. I felt dismayed that I had "sandbagged" my chief with a case far out of his area of expertise. He graciously stated that it was a fine learning experience and never seemed to hold it against me for this rather cruel trick on him.

Even more amazing, he called me into his office that spring and told me that Dr. Seymour Gray, the chief of the gastrointestinal division, was stepping down and asked if I would consider taking his place. I explained that I had no special training in intestinal, liver or pancreatic diseases, but he said, "There is nothing special about this field that a well-trained internist cannot master." After discussions with my wife, Warren Wacker and Bert Vallee, I agreed to begin a new job as Chief of Gastroenterology in July 1963.

9

Chief of Gastroenterology

◆

1963–1968

I became Chief of Gastroenterology on July 5, 1963, after a two-week vacation in Maine. I replaced Dr. Seymour Gray, a gastroenterologist who trained in Chicago and served at the Brigham for almost twenty years. Dr. Gray never focused on any one area of research, but changed from one popular topic to another throughout his career. As a result, he never made an important mark in gastrointestinal research. Because of the reputation of the Peter Bent Brigham he did attract a few excellent fellows. In spite of little help from him they achieved some important publications. Two whom I knew were Robert Donaldson and Donald Ostrow, who went on to have successful careers. When I took over, there was only one fellow in gastroenterology, Americo Abbruzzese. Americo was raised in Lynn, Massachusetts, where as a football star he obtained a scholarship to Union College in New York State. Unfortunately, his grades were not good enough to get into a U.S. medical school. So he looked abroad and was admitted to the medical school in Florence, Italy, made possible because he was fluent in Italian. He considered these four years among the most enjoyable of his life. He returned to the United States for an internship at Lynn Hospital and residency at Creighton University Medical School in Omaha, Nebraska. As a resident he became ill with the flu and began taking many aspirin tablets. He soon developed black tarry stools and vomited some blood. When he was admitted to the hospital the doctors did a blood count and a blood smear. The chief of hematology came to his room and told him that the blood smear showed that he had acute myelogenous leukemia, which in those days was a sentence of death within three to four weeks. After Americo considered his imminent death for 12 hours, the next morning the hematologist told him that they had mixed up the blood smears between himself and a patient with leukemia and that his smear was normal. It turned out that the aspirin had caused gastritis or a stomach ulcer which caused the bleeding. This experience had a profound effect on Americo and he never forgot what it was like to be a patient and be given information about a life-endangering disease. He always had great empathy for people he cared for.

Americo learned from Seymour Gray to do upper endoscopy with the semirigid Schindler gastroscope, which was a metal shaft with a flexible tip and internal mirrors. Getting it down the esophagus into the patient's stomach required something like sword swallowing. I needed an endoscopist and someone to teach me how to do endoscopy. Americo was an honest, modest, hard-working, caring physician, always cheerful. I liked him a great deal and asked him to be my assistant chief of gastroenterology. He and I were appointed as Associates in Medicine at the Brigham and I was named Associate at Harvard Medical School, which is the bottom rung of the academic ladder.

I set out to train myself in the specialty of gastroenterology because I had never had any formal training. When I was consulted on a patient with a gastrointestinal disease, I did a complete history and physical examination and then I went to the Harvard Medical School Library and read up on what I thought the patient's problem was. I then wrote my consultation note and gave recommendations. I read all the textbooks on gastroenterology. One of them was considered the "bible" of our specialty, written by a Dr. Bockus and his associates in Philadelphia. I found that it was almost entirely anecdotal, consisting of clinical opinions, little of it being based on good clinical research. Kurt Isselbacher, who had been my senior resident when I was a fourth-year student at Massachusetts General Hospital, took over as Chief of Gastroenterology there. He was never trained in gastroenterology and did his research in biochemistry at the National Institutes of Health. We discussed the fact that neither of us had been trained in the subject, It was his opinion, as it was Dr. Thorn's, that gastroenterology was not yet a scientific discipline and it was up to people like us to make it such.

Shortly after I took over the position, Dr. Francis Moore called me into his office. He said that he was pleased that I had been given the appointment and that we could work together to make medical and surgical gastroenterology at the Brigham outstanding. His idea was that I would function like the gastrointestinal physicians at the Lahey Clinic and find cases for his surgeons to operate upon. I went to Dr. Thorn and told him about this discussion. He said that I should do what I thought was best academically for myself and for the division. He also commented that "Franny" was not running the Department of Medicine at the Brigham.

I was surprised to learn that most of the chiefs of gastroenterology in the main Boston hospitals had never trained formally in the subject. I already mentioned Kurt Isselbacher at MGH. Franz Ingelfinger, a senior person in the field and Chief of Medicine and Gastroenterology at Boston University School of Medicine, was self-taught. James F. Patterson, the chief of gastroenterology at Tufts Medical School, was also self-trained. The only chief who had been trained in gastroenterology was Norman Zamchek, who directed the Harvard Service at Boston City Hospital. Charles Davidson was chief of the liver section at the Harvard Service at Boston City Hospital and he also was self-trained. Thomas Chalmers, an internist on the Harvard Service at Boston City Hospital, founded a cooperative research group among all the Boston hospitals called the Boston Inter-Hospital Liver Group in order to do controlled clinical trials on liver disease and its treatment. These people played a major role among those who helped bring gastroenterology into the modern era.

I was greatly impressed in my reading by the controlled clinical trials which were being pioneered in England by George Pickering and Stanley Peart on hypertension at St. Mary's Hospital in London and by Richard Doll in the dietary treatment of ulcer disease. Dr. Doll was not a gastroenterologist but rather an internist and early epidemiologist at Oxford. The Chief of Gastroenterology at Oxford, Dr. Sidney Truelove, was also doing excellent controlled trials on the treatment of inflammatory bowel disease. After being in charge for one year, I was asked to give a grand rounds on peptic ulcer disease. I read from the "bible" texts according to Bockus and then debunked the traditional six-meal bland diet with milk and cream. I described the new findings from England which showed that the diet had no effect on the healing of ulcers. The faculty, the dieticians and the senior practitioners who attended grand rounds were quite upset by my talk. They said "What should we do? Are we supposed to feed these people a normal diet?" Weak evidence was available for healing of ulcers using new antacids that were made from magnesium and aluminum hydroxides. After my grand rounds talk the Brigham staff gradually gave up the traditional ulcer diets.

Americo and I were unhappy with the semi-rigid gastroscope so we bought the first fiber-optic endoscope, manufactured by American Cystoscope Makers Inc. We taught ourselves to use it by trying it on our patients. The original optics were poor but each year they came out with a new and better model. The Japanese soon led in this field and Olympus was the best manufacturer. We would tell Olympus that we were willing to test their new endoscope and if we found it satisfactory, we would tell them so and then keep it as a gift. We were soon able to enter the duodenum with these new scopes and see duodenal ulcers, which no one had been able to do before. The function of the upper endoscope was almost entirely for diagnosis. There was no endoscopic treatment available in those early years. If patients had a massive bleed from the upper gastrointestinal tract, their management required cooperation among the house staff, the gastroenterologist, the surgeons and the radiologist. Surgery was our last resort to stop bleeding from an ulcer. Which operation was best caused great surgical controversies. Francis Moore was a pioneer in doing vagotomy, cutting the main vagus nerve which stimulated acid production in the stomach, and he remained interested in the problem of peptic ulcer. Eventually, the operation vagotomy and antrectomy, cutting the vagus nerve and removing the far end of the stomach called the antrum, became the standard procedure for a stomach or duodenal ulcer. It was less crippling than removing two-thirds to three-quarters of the stomach and the recurrence of ulcers was low. Still there were many unpleasant side effects. All of this changed when the first histamine-2 blockers were developed in the 1980s, the first effective drugs to heal ulcers. New endoscopes allowed cautery of vessels in bleeding ulcers. Surgery for peptic ulcer disease was rarely done thereafter.

I decided to focus on pancreatic diseases because no one else was doing this in Boston and I had a great interest in the pancreas from a biochemical point of view. I wanted to improve the methods for the diagnoses of acute pancreatitis, chronic pancreatitis, and cancer of the pancreas. I taught myself to do pancreatic function tests. These required placing a tube through the mouth into the stomach, through the stomach and into the duodenum, stimulating pancreatic secretion with the hormones secretin and/or pancreozymin, collecting the juice from the duodenum and analyzing the enzyme activities and bicarbonate concentrations. When patients needed pancreatic surgery I called upon Dr. John Brooks, one of our best general surgeons, and upon other general surgeons who had an interest in pancreatic disease. We had an excellent nuclear medicine department which pioneered in doing radioseleno-methionine scans of the pancreas, which gave us a rough picture of the gland and occasionally allowed us to see a tumor. We embarked on a major effort toward the early diagnosis of cancer of the pancreas, which was 95 percent fatal when discovered late. When we discovered a small tumor, Dr. Brooks would carry out a total removal of the pancreas in an attempt to prevent recurrences. The patients, of course, became insulin-dependent diabetics and had to be fed pancreatic enzymes by mouth to digest their food. We took part in their long-term care. Eventually, Dr. Brooks published 33 cases with resectable ductal pancreatic cancer and total removal of the pancreas, with an operative mortality of 12 percent but five-year survivals of only 15 percent. Other centers also published similar results and total pancreatectomy was abandoned except in rare cases. We thought that our failures were due to lack of better early diagnostic methods. In spite of many years of effort using all the new imaging tests and many variations in surgery, the mortality from cancer of the pancreas still remains 90 to 95 percent overall and the survival time averages around six months.

I discussed with Dr. Vallee and Warren Wacker what area of research I should choose and what topic I should use to apply for a National Institutes of Health research grant. In 1963, these grants were relatively easy to obtain compared to later in the 1970s and 1980s. Dr. Vallee suggested that I continue studies of isolated mitochondria in Warburg flasks which had been published from his laboratory. His study showed that carbon tetrachloride uncoupled oxidative phosphorylation, i.e., oxygen consumption no longer led to production of high energy phosphate compounds in mitochondria, and caused uptake of calcium into and loss of potassium from the mitochondria, leading to cell energy failure and death of the cells. We agreed that I should test other halogenated hydrocarbons, especially those being used in medicine as anesthetics. I reviewed the carbon tetrachloride literature and found that it affected not only mitochondria but all parts of the liver cell including the cytoplasmic membrane, the smooth and rough endoplasmic reticulum and the nucleus of the cells. Thus it damaged and interfered with functions far beyond the mitochondria. My grant application entitled "Chlorinated hydrocarbon intoxication as a model in studies of liver disease" was funded by the gastrointestinal section of the National Institutes of Health of the Public Health Service.

My first technician was Marta Piras from Argentina, the wife of a fellow in the Biophysics lab. She had a master's degree in biochemistry and was a skillful worker, although quite temperamental. We used an instrument called a Warburg apparatus, which we borrowed from the Biophysics lab. We learned to measure oxidative-phosphorylation by mitochondria after isolating them by differential centrifugation of liver homogenates. Using the Warburg flasks was technically very difficult. Their manometer levels, which contained air and liquid, had to be read every minute in each of 10 flasks as the oxygen was consumed by the mitochondria. We removed the carbon dioxide produced by the mitochondria by an acid trap centered in the flask. We tipped in various reagents from little side tubes and looked at their effects on oxygen consumption. At the end of the procedure, we stopped all reactions with acid and analyzed how much phosphorus had been removed, presumably as high energy phosphate compounds like adenosine triphosphate (ATP). Otto Warburg in Germany and Hans Krebs in England, who pioneered the use of this apparatus to measure cell respiration, certainly won my respect when I learned to use these instruments. Later on, the oxygen consumption was measured quickly and easily with an oxygen electrode and the manometers no longer were necessary.

Marta and I looked at a series of hydrocarbons containing chlorine (Cl), bromine (Br), or fluorine (F) and found in isolated mitochondria that many of these compounds injured the mitochondria as did carbon tetrachloride. At this time, a new anesthetic was developed called halothane, whose formula was $CF_3CHBrCl$. As an anesthetic it was a major improvement over anything previously available but some patients who were exposed repeatedly to halothane developed massive liver necrosis and died. We found in the flasks with mitochondria that halothane uncoupled (disconnected) oxidation from formation of high energy phosphate at all three coupling sites in the mitochondria, caused irreversible swelling of the mitochondria and caused loss of potassium. We found that chloroform ($CHCl_3$), carbon tetrachloride, benzene and diethyl ether all uncoupled the mitochondria in the flasks, and that it was a function of their relative oil/water solubility ratios. Carbon tetrachloride being the most lipid-soluble was the most injurious. However, when we gave halothane to intact rats, put them to sleep for hours, repeated the treatment many times and then isolated their mitochondria, we could find no injury. We published the effects of halothane and other hydrocarbons on the isolated mitochondria in the journal *Biochemistry* in 1966. Years later, it was found that halothane is metabolized by the cytochrome P450 enzymes of the liver to form free radicals that bind to proteins. These modified proteins act as antigens and cause an immune reaction. The liver cells which contained these antigens on their surface were then destroyed by the body's immune cells.

I went on to study the effects of carbon tetrachloride on the tubular membrane system in the cell which manufactures proteins, metabolizes drugs and contains a large number of drug metabolizing enzymes called the cytochrome P450 family. My studies yielded no important results so I gave up on studying halogenated hydrocarbons. Shortly thereafter the P450 enzymes in liver became a hot research topic, which continues to this very day. However, I decided to change to a new research area, the urea cycle enzymes of liver and their inducers and suppressors.

The surgical service had a funded fellowship for a surgical trainee to come from St. Mary's Hospital in London to work at the Brigham but they had no candidate for 1964–1965. I was asked if I would like to train a medical person in my laboratory using their George Gorham Peters Fellowship. After discussing candidates with the chief of medicine at St. Mary's Hospital, we arranged to have a well-trained internist named David Parry come over to do research in my laboratory. David had trained at many English hospitals but had not been able to obtain a consultantship, which is the highest level of internal medicine in the British national health system. He needed a "BTB" (Been to Boston) degree, especially a research experience which often helped "Brits" obtain a consultant position. He did not want to do clinical gastroenterology, just work in the laboratory. I had already begun investigating the use of the ornithine transcarbamylase assay in serum as a liver function test because OTC, as this urea cycle enzyme is abbreviated, is found only in the liver and to a smaller extent in the intestines. The assays which had previously been used were tedious and not reproducible. David Parry and I worked out an assay in serum and in mitochondria where we simply added the substrates in the way the enzyme encountered them in the mitochondria. We defined optimal concentrations of carbamyl phosphate and ornithine, optimal pH and buffers to control pH, in order to form citrulline and phosphate. We assayed citrulline by a sensitive colorimetric method and made the overall assay sensitive enough to detect OTC in normal serum where the activity was extremely low. We also found that serum OTC activities increased 10- to 100-fold when there was liver injury. We concluded that OTC was the best available liver-specific serum enzyme assay and began measuring it as a new test for Brigham hospital patients. David and I published a paper reporting his work in the *Journal of Laboratory and Clinical Medicine* in 1969. When David went back to England, he was appointed as a consultant in medicine at the Birmingham Regional Hospital in Sutton-Coldfield. We remained close friends and I visited him twice in England. At the age of 45, David died suddenly of an acute heart attack while shoveling snow. I did not know that he had a strong family history of coronary artery disease and that he had had warning signs of heart pain. I and my family grieved along with his wife and children for this tragic loss of such a lovable person and fine physician.

    The first clinical fellow who worked under my tutelage was Russell Jeffrey, in 1964–1965. He had finished a year of senior residency at the Beth Israel Hospital, one of the Harvard teaching hospitals, and was already an excellent internist. He learned to do upper endoscopy, working with Americo and using our new fiber-optic upper endoscopes. He helped me do a study of magnesium deficiency and learned to measure magnesium on a flame spectrometer that was built in the Biophysics Laboratory. After one year, he went into practice in Wakefield, Massachusetts, near his birthplace doing general internal medicine and some gastroenterology. He continued to practice there until retirement, always taking his turn on nights and weekends staffing the intensive care units where he had to deal with severe cardiac, pulmonary, and infectious disease and gastrointestinal problems.

Claude Thomas "Tom" Nuzum came to see me in 1963 when he was a fourth-year Harvard medical student, and asked if he could do a research project in my laboratory. My grandmother was named Cynthia Jane Nuzum Snodgrass and I asked if we could by any chance be related. He had an elderly aunt in West Virginia who had written a book on the Nuzum family describing all the descendants of "Black Dick" Nuzum, who came from Northern Ireland around 1770 and set up a mill in West Virginia, where he ground corn and made whiskey. He had a large family and one of his sons, George, moved to Zanesville, Ohio, and produced eighteen children with his wife, Sophie. These were our common ancestors, one branch of George's family going to Kentucky, Tom's branch, and the other to Wisconsin, my branch. Tom and I were fourth cousins. I set him to work testing the old published assay for OTC which he showed was useless. He began to develop a new one, work which was later carried on by David Parry. After Tom finished his internship and residency at the University of Kentucky Medical Center in Lexington, he returned to my laboratory as a research fellow from 1966 through 1969. He led the effort to improve the assays of all five urea cycle enzymes. He scaled them down so that all five assays could be done on 10 to 20 mg of wet liver tissue, making it possible to assess urea cycle enzyme status on a needle biopsy. He arranged to work with Sarah Ratner at the Public Health Research Institute in New York City. Dr. Ratner had shown that the urea cycle discovered by Hans Krebs, which he described as ornithine to citrulline to arginine to urea, a three-step reaction, was actually a five-step reaction. She showed that citrulline and aspartic acid were combined by an enzyme to make a double amino acid called argininosuccinate and this was then split to arginine and fumarate by a second enzyme. Arginine was split to urea and ornithine as Krebs knew, restarting the cycle. Ratner also did major work on the first enzyme of the cycle, carbamyl phosphate synthetase, which formed a compound, carbamyl phosphate, from ammonia, bicarbonate and ATP. Carbamyl phosphate reacts with ornithine to form citrulline, catalyzed by OTC. With her help, Tom and I learned to make partly purified rat liver OTC and beef liver argininosuccinase, which were necessary as coupling enzymes in our assays. Arginase was commercially available. Thus we had the ability to make coupled enzyme reactions of all five urea cycle enzymes, measuring in the first two enzymes the formation of citrulline and in the last three enzymes the release of urea. We published these methods under the title "Multiple assays of the five urea cycle enzymes in human liver homogenates" in a book called *The Urea Cycle,* published in 1976. Tom had made sure that the conditions for our assays of these five enzymes were optimal in the human liver for their pH, substrates, buffers and cofactors. These methods were soon used worldwide and continue to be so used unless people feel that they need to use radioactive substrates, which allow more sensitivity but are more cumbersome to carry out.

Tom and I demonstrated that the urea cycle enzymes in monkey livers adapted to the level of dietary protein as they did in rats. At the New England Regional Primate Center, we took turns tube-feeding two species of macaques a high protein liquid diet for two weeks, biopsied their livers and repeated the process with a low protein diet. Tom assayed the enzymes. After this successful experiment, Tom and I consumed a diet containing 400 grams of protein per day for two weeks. Then we collected our pancreatic juice from a tube in the duodenum after stimulation of the pancreas with the hormones secretin and pancreozymin. Next we consumed a synthetic diet containing only one gram of protein per day with equal calorie content to the high protein diet and collected pancreatic juice again. We assayed the pancreatic enzymes and showed that the protein-digesting enzymes in human juice did not increase on the high versus the low protein diet as they do in rats. After each diet period I convinced Americo against his better judgment to perform a needle biopsy of my liver and Tom assayed my urea cycle enzymes on both specimens. The human enzymes all increased on the high versus the low protein diets but not as much as they did in monkeys. The journal *Science* published in 1971 the paper entitled "Urea cycle enzyme adaption to dietary protein in primates," authored by Nuzum and Snodgrass. I deleted the results of my liver enzyme responses because I was shamed by my wife, Bert Vallee and Americo for ever undergoing the somewhat risky liver biopsies.

Tom stayed on at the Brigham in 1969–70 as a senior resident. He then went to the University of Kentucky Medical School as an assistant professor and later to the University of North Carolina School of Medicine and became associate professor. He worked in the gastroenterology division and in the dean's office as a supervisor of student off-campus programs until his retirement. Tom did no more laboratory research but became a good gastrointestinal clinician, specializing in liver disease and later in liver transplantation.

We have remained close friends throughout these years. Tom had been captain of the Harvard varsity heavyweight crew in college and in 1967, while in my laboratory, he convinced me to join the Cambridge Boat Club and resume our rowing, but this time in single shells. We both rowed our first Head of the Charles Regatta in 1968 as novices. I have continued sculling and racing throughout my life, most recently completing my thirteenth Head of the Charles race in 2004. Tom's son Henry subsequently captained the Harvard heavyweight varsity crew and later rowed a double shell in the finals of the 2000 and 2004 Olympic regattas, coming in sixth both times.

In 1963, I took the boards of internal medicine exams, both written and oral, and passed them. Then I began to see private patients in the late afternoon when I had finished clinical and research duties in the hospital. Most of the patients I saw were referred from other doctors as consultations. I never wanted to develop a large private practice but only to help patients by doing problem-solving consultations and sending the patients back to their regular doctors, who would give them their ongoing care. This practice resulted in a small supplement to my salary, which was set in the first year at $13,000 a year, derived from supervising the hospital chemistry lab, serving as director of a general medical clinic one half-day a week, helping Dr. Warren Wacker in a liver clinic one half-day a week and serving as assistant director of the new clinical research center. I requested no salary from my research grants but assigned all funds to my technicians, supplies and equipment. I was able to bill private patients for consultations on the hospital wards and for procedures such as upper endoscopies, liver biopsies or pancreatic function tests. This was the way Dr. Thorn pieced together an income for his staff physicians because there was no salary line for doctors at the Brigham. Although he was the Hersey Professor of the Theory and Practice of Physic, this famous professorship at Harvard Medical School carried few endowment funds and he had to earn his own salary from private practice. When the Samuel A. Levine endowed professorship was established at the Brigham, Dr. Thorn appointed himself as the first incumbent so that, as he told me, "Harvard would at last pay part of my salary."

In 1967, I decided to take the board of internal medicine exams in gastroenterology because they had a rule that fellows who trained with me needed to have their mentor be boarded in order for them to obtain their gastroenterology boards. The exam that year was to be held at Mayo Clinic, all day on a Saturday. Dr. Franz Ingelfinger, who was coauthor with me on a chapter on the pancreas in Harrison's textbook of medicine, was on the board of examiners and because he knew me and worked with me, he had to recuse himself. He advised me that the oral examiners would expect me to be able to consult upon or manage patients in any area of gastroenterology or liver disease. I spent the previous six months reading all of the textbooks of gastroenterology so that I would know the "party line" to give to the examiners. I focused on areas that I knew little about, especially esophageal, gastric and small intestinal motility and inflammatory bowel diseases. Dr. Ingelfinger said the board was unhappy because I had never done any formal training in gastroenterology. George Thorn was able to convince them to let me take the test anyway. Dr. Ingelfinger told me privately that one of the Mayo examiners was "out to get that chief resident of George Thorn." The night before the exam in Rochester, Minnesota, I was so anxious that I could not sleep so I got up and went to a movie.

The examination format consisted of eight one-hour oral or practical exams, each time before a new team of two examiners. The first team happened to include a person who had been one of my teachers at Massachusetts General Hospital. He and his partner asked me to discuss carbon tetrachloride poisoning. I explained that it was not a fair question because it was my research topic. They said that I should go ahead anyway and tell them what I knew, so I gave them a one-hour lecture on all the knowledge that I had written into my grant applications. The next team gave me a patient who had been followed at Mayo Clinic since the 1920s for duodenal ulcer disease. He had every complication of this disease, many surgeries and the complications of these surgeries. I had a half-hour to do the workup and then a half-hour to present my findings. This patient was a cooperative and knowledgeable Swedish man who gave me an excellent summary of his 40-year history in a short time. I did a complete history and physical examination and among my findings, I detected a nodule in his thyroid gland. When I presented my findings, the Mayo Clinic records did not mention a thyroid nodule and the Mayo clinic staff examiner was quite upset that they had missed it. It could have been a parathyroid tumor, which was known to cause severe peptic ulcer disease.

Then the next hour was a "practicum," interpreting tissue slides under a microscope, esophageal motility tracings, photographs of skin lesions and pictures of findings during upper endoscopy. Then there were more case discussions. At the end of the day, they told us who had passed. Surprisingly, I passed with flying colors and one of the examiners told Dr. Ingelfinger that the chief resident of Thorn was "amazing." So much for formal training! One man failed the exam because he only examined the abdomen. Thus it was true when Dr. Thorn told me that good internal medicine training is essential to being a good specialist.

George Thorn was one of six editors of Harrison's textbook of medicine, the newest and soon most popular textbook of medicine in the world. Franz Ingelfinger, who was then Professor of Medicine at Boston University and head of their gastroenterology division, wrote the chapters on the pancreas and on the gallbladder and bile ducts. He was then appointed as chief editor of the *New England Journal of Medicine,* so he asked to be relieved of the textbook responsibility. Dr. Thorn suggested that I coauthor the chapter on the pancreas in the fifth edition

(1966) and then in the sixth edition take the chapter over myself. I enjoyed working with Dr. Ingelfinger as we updated the chapter on the pancreas. I also wrote a short "Approach to the diagnosis of pancreatic disease." He was critical and liked to put down conventional wisdom when there was nothing to back it up. He taught me that every statement in a textbook chapter must be backed up by good studies and references, a policy that I continued the rest of my chapter-writing days. For the sixth edition in 1970, I obtained permission to write a short section entitled "Biochemistry and physiology of the exocrine pancreas." I believed that many of the readers needed an update on these topics because they had not heard anything about this material since they were in medical school and could not understand the rest of the chapter on the testing of pancreatic function or the clinical sections without a basic review. This section was a big success and in the seventh edition in 1974, Drs. David Alpers and Kurt Isselbacher from Massachusetts General added a basic science introduction to their section on liver diseases. Kurt also asked me to take on the chapters on the gallbladder and bile ducts in the sixth edition. When I pleaded no special knowledge of this area, he said, "You just had a gallbladder attack and had it removed; therefore you can speak from personal experience." I asked that Americo Abbruzzese be my coauthor to help me in looking up this new literature and writing the chapters. He translated a good part of Harrison's textbook into Italian and that edition sold well. We began the new chapter with "Physiology of the biliary system and chemistry of the bile," a topic that was new and exciting because of the research by Dr. Donald Small and his colleagues at Boston University. By the eighth edition in 1977, most of the organ system disease chapters included a basic science section to introduce the chapters. Because Harrison's textbook was used throughout the world, my reputation as an expert in pancreatic and biliary disease far exceeded my reputation in the field of urea cycle enzymes and diseases with high blood ammonia levels. I always considered carefully what I wrote in those chapters because someone, somewhere would take that book off the shelf and rely on what I said about the diagnosis and treatment of his individual patient. After I moved to Indianapolis and George Thorn was no longer an editor, Kurt Isselbacher, editor-in-chief for the ninth edition, replaced me with people he had trained at Massachusetts General. This is the way multi-authored textbooks are written. I was pleased to see that the chapters on the biliary tree, gallbladder and pancreas still began with basic science reviews. My final effort in the field of textbook chapters was to write the "Pathophysiology of the pancreas" in *Sodeman's Pathologic Physiology*, in both the sixth and seventh editions in 1979 and 1985.

The next three clinical and research fellows who trained with me at the Brigham were Martin Sarner, Stephen Curtis, and Mordekhai Moritz. Martin Sarner was a student of Professor Stanley Peart at St. Mary's Hospital and the University of London Medical School. Dr. Peart recommended him as a bright and energetic physician. Others said that he was an occasionally abrasive young man. I found him to be as described but never abrasive. Everyone at the Brigham liked him and that included most of the surgeons. He did his research on the effect of magnesium deficiency of rats on their exocrine pancreatic function. Unfortunately he found no impairment of function even with near-lethal magnesium deficiency. He also worked on a perfused rabbit pancreas model with a friend he made at the Harvard dental school. He learned endoscopy from Americo Abbruzzese and helped me organize a popular medical-surgical gastrointestinal conference at noon on Thursdays.

Harvard medical students regularly elected to take our course, medical-surgical gastroenterology, taught by our group and by John Brooks, a gastrointestinal surgeon. They examined gastrointestinal patients from the time of referral to the Brigham, helped us come to a diagnosis, scrubbed in during the surgery and helped care for the patients postoperatively. Some of our course graduates became famous academic surgeons.

Martin met an Israeli woman who was working for her PhD at Harvard Medical School with Professor Luigi Perini, a pioneer molecular biologist. Perini had sheltered her family in Italy and protected them from the Fascists. Martin and Nitza were married in a traditional Jewish wedding in Brookline and then they spent their honeymoon camping all over the United States in their Volvo station wagon. Martin finished three years at the Brigham and then went to England and was awarded a consultant position in gastroenterology at Portsmouth Hospital on the south coast. He later moved to London as a consultant and Chief of Gastroenterology at University College Hospital and Medical School and built a unit of outstanding people, eventually joining with the group at Middlesex Hospital. He served as a dean of the University College Medical School and as secretary of the British Pancreatic Association. He has always been one of my best friends and supporters. In 1972, he came to Boston for six weeks to help me teach the new gastrointestinal course in the Harvard-MIT Program in Health Sciences and Technology. We traded our house in Indianapolis for his house in London so that his three daughters could see the United States and Woody and I could get to know England and Scotland. After three daughters, he and Nitza had a son. We often met at GI meetings in the United States and especially in Chicago each November for the American Pancreatic Association meetings.

Stephen Curtis interned at the Brigham in 1963–64 and was a junior resident in 1964–65. He came from the University of Iowa and I knew from his work on our house staff that he was an intelligent, hard-working man with leadership ability. He asked to join our laboratory because he wanted a career in academic gastroenterology. He became an excellent clinician and skillful endoscopist. I assigned him a research project to identify enzymes found only or mostly in liver cells, derived from different subcellular fractions of the liver cell such as the cytoplasm, mitochondria, lysosomes, endoplasmic reticulum (ER) and nuclei. We used carbon tetrachloride as a model form of liver injury in rats and followed the serum and liver fraction activities of these chosen enzymes over time. Steve found enzymes that were relatively specific for these fractions of liver. We hoped that the increases and time courses of serum enzymes would reflect different types of liver injury, serving as a "biochemical biopsy." Our other model to compare with carbon tetrachloride was bile duct ligation.

Steve was efficient and an excellent worker in the laboratory and skillful at supervising technicians. When it came to writing up results for his paper, however, he developed writer's block. Finally, I wrote the paper myself. The results were quite interesting. He found an enzyme quite specific for the cytoplasm in liver, sorbitol dehydrogenase. He used our urea cycle enzyme, ornithine transcarbamylase, as the quite specific liver mitochondrial enzyme. Steve found a drug that was split only by a liver microsomal esterase to test for the smooth ER. Two other enzymes found in the lysosomes and nuclei were not specific for liver cells. The serum cytoplasmic enzyme increased within three hours after carbon tetrachloride given orally to rats and the mitochondrial enzymes appeared in the serum at 6 hours but the microsomal enzyme did not appear until 23 hours, although we knew that damage to the ER occurred very early. Lysosomal and nuclear enzymes never appeared in the serum. There was no correlation between the activities in the liver cell fractions with the serum activities except for the microsomal esterase, which was decreased in the liver and elevated in serum at 24 hours. The idea of a "biochemical biopsy" in serum did not look feasible as a result of Steve's work. After the two year fellowship, Steve became a senior resident in 1967–68 and then George Thorn chose him as the chief medical resident in 1968–69. He excelled at both jobs. He was recruited back to Iowa as assistant professor of medicine in their GI department but his life-long asthma flared up and he then moved to Palms Springs, California to practice. He later trained in radiology, particularly GI radiology, and has been very successful as a practicing radiologist and gastroenterologist.

Mordekhai Moritz is an Israeli who went to medical school in Geneva, Switzerland. He did his clinical training in the Beilinson Hospital in Israel. Then he came to the United States and did one year of clinical gastroenterology at Yale in 1966–67. He wanted research experience, so he joined us in 1967–68. He was an excellent clinician and became skilled at endoscopy. He joined Steve Curtis on the project on serum enzymes in model forms of liver injury. He did the bile duct ligations and supervised the technician. He helped me write up the two papers. The cytoplasmic and mitochondrial enzymes in serum rose in one hour and peaked at 24 hours and they never correlated with the activities in the liver cell fractions. We concluded that it must be retention of certain bile salts that injures the liver cells, particularly the cell membrane and the mitochondrial membrane early. The results did differ from those with carbon tetrachloride. We published two papers in the journal *Gastroenterology* in 1972, entitled "Serum enzymes derived from liver cell fractions. 1. The response to carbon tetrachloride intoxication in rats and 2. Responses to bile duct ligation in rats." Comments from my peers were that these papers were well done and quite sophisticated but were no breakthrough in interpreting serum enzyme changes in liver injury. "Moti," as we called him, then went to Tufts Medical School in 1968–69 in their gastrointestinal division to work on ulcerative colitis. During 1969–1970 he took a fellowship at the Lemuel Shattuck Hospital in Boston to work on small bowel transport. Then he was made assistant professor of medicine at Temple University Medical School, Philadelphia, in their gastrointestinal division but after three years he tired of academic life and went into practice in Scranton, Pennsylvania, where he became a successful and well-to-do practitioner, specializing in endoscopy. Moti went from place to place looking for what he wanted to do and finally realized that it was to take care of patients, not to do research.

I became a member of the American Gastroenterology Association in 1965 and a Fellow of the American College of Physicians in 1968. I was honored to be accepted into the American Society of Biological Chemistry and the American Institute of Nutrition in 1968, probably because of the recommendations from Bert Vallee, my research mentor. Belonging to these societies is like getting your union card.

We added a fourth daughter to our family in December, 1965. Emily almost did not make it because Woody fell down our cellar steps in October. This fall precipitated premature labor. It took medications and six weeks of bed rest to get Emily to term. She got so much mothering from her three sisters that her first sentence was "leader lone" (leave her alone).

Through 1968, our program attracted good fellows and had an excellent clinical reputation at the Brigham but caused no big impact from our biochemical research. I failed to take advantage of the clinical research center to do clinical investigations that might make the major clinical journals. I had no excuse not to do this because I was the assistant director of the CRC under Warren Wacker and in 1969 became its program director. Meanwhile, George Cahill, my old intern partner, and his team from the Joslin Clinic did major studies on metabolic responses to fasting in obese humans in our clinical center.

In 1967, at a site visit of my training program, Professor Myron Brin, a professor of nutrition, told me that John Halver, the director of the Western Fish and Nutrition Laboratory in Cook, Washington, was always looking for people to help him in his studies on salmon. I had long had an idea that the reason that Pacific salmon spawn and then die was that they had exhausted all of their stores of fat and muscle in their long migration without food from the ocean to the fresh water spawning grounds. I postulated that they died of energy depletion and cellular ion leakage. I thought we would see failure of cells to maintain normal levels of potassium and magnesium on the inside and the ability to keep sodium and calcium out of the cells because of failure of energy production, particularly ATP. John Halver funded a truck camper for me which we drove from Boston to his laboratory on the Columbia River, along with my wife and four children, including our new fourth daughter Emily who was then 1-1/2 years old and still in diapers. In the laboratory, we collected samples of plasma, red cells, brain, heart, skeletal muscle, liver, kidney and gills from juvenile salmon in their fish hatchery. The species was king salmon, *Oncorhynchus tshawytscha*. We froze the tissue specimens on dry ice. Then we went to a laboratory on the coast at Bowman's Bay, where we were able to adapt the same small salmon weighing about 60 to 100 grams to seawater by increasing the percentage of seawater by 20% each day over 5 days and then leaving them in seawater for 9 days to see what happened during this major stress which salmon undergo when they move from fresh to seawater. We also collected tissues from mature salmon caught at sea on their way to spawn.

We then collected tissue from spawning adults in a fish hatchery pool after six months in fresh water without food, by which time they were emaciated and covered with a fungus growth.

We took these specimens back to the Brigham and analyzed them for sodium, potassium, magnesium, calcium and nitrogen. Amazingly, the spawning, dying salmon had a normal body composition of these cations in their tissues and no rise in tissue sodium or calcium. The only abnormality was in the juveniles after adaptation to seawater, where the potassium per gram of nitrogen decreased in many tissues but they still appeared healthy. It surprised all who took part in this study how capable salmon were in maintaining normal cation composition through these stressful changes from no sodium in fresh water to high sodium in seawater and back to fresh water again plus starvation. No evidence for adrenal exhaustion or "pump" failure was seen. I received more reprint requests for this paper in *Comparative Biochemistry and Physiology* (1971) than any other paper I ever wrote because there was a worldwide interest in salmon throughout the Northern hemispheres. People read about and did research on salmon in the United States, Canada, Japan, the USSR, Norway, Sweden, Iceland and Scotland. John Halver later became professor and director of fish research at the University of Washington in Seattle and retired with many honors and a worldwide reputation. My regret is that we have seen so little of John and his wife and children, and only keep up through Christmas letters.

George Thorn continued to add jobs and responsibilities upon my shoulders. Although I gave up directing the Brigham chemistry lab to a colleague of Bert Vallee's, I continued to work Tuesday evenings doing counseling in the alcoholism clinic until 1964. Dr. Thorn reorganized the medical outpatient clinics partly at my urging and created day and evening clinics, staffed by general internists, house staff and medical specialists all doing general internal medicine. A clinic director was expected to meet with all the physicians to help with problems outside their usual specialties and to have a conference at the end of every clinic day to discuss problem patients. I directed the Thursday afternoon clinic, and Americo Abbruzzese the Saturday morning clinic. The house staff warmly welcomed the change, but our specialists hated it. Cardiologists and hematologists had to do internal medicine and also staff their specialty clinics. I recall teaching Bernard Lown, my former teacher of EKG and cardiology, how to palpate a spleen. This job lasted from 1964 to 1967 and ended when the specialists rose up in unison and convinced Dr. Thorn to release them from doing general medicine duty.

I served as assistant director of the clinical research center from 1963 to 1967 and, when Warren Wacker became ill, as program director from 1967 to 1973. This required me to make daily rounds with the nurses, do problem solving and, most burdensome, to write the annual reports. The investigators gave me poorly written and documented summaries and I had to make them shine so we could continue our funding. The grant renewals in 1968 and 1973 each totaled about 600 pages.

I greatly enjoyed giving lectures on the pancreas, gallbladder and bile ducts each year in the second-year pathophysiology course at Harvard Medical School.

I was also a laboratory section leader in the course teaching with Professor Tom Wilson, chairman of the Department of Physiology, and Dr. Franz von Lichtenburg, a pathologist and friend from the Brigham. I wrote up cases for the students and we discussed the pertinent basic science, pathology and clinical care in an integrated fashion. The students took turns discussing these cases. One student always sat in the back of the room and read, or hid, behind the *New York Times*. He was very smart and knew the cases when called on but obviously had other interests beside medical school. Michael Crichton was his name and he went on to write novels based on medical or scientific topics, which became best-sellers. His novels were then made into popular movies.

My teaching load grew yearly: third-year medicine instructor; lecturer on gastrointestinal diseases at the Brigham course on advances on internal medicine yearly; grand rounds twice yearly; a yearly GI medical-surgical course in Maine; attending physician on the medical wards twice yearly; and attending on GI consultations six months a year. The clinical load in GI was heavy. Americo and I took turns staffing consults and procedures, mostly upper endoscopies, every other month as well as rounding with the fellows and the fourth-year students who elected our course in gastroenterology. I performed 500 liver biopsies during 1964–1972. We then covered for each other for vacations—Americo took off in July and I took off during August—and we covered for each other when we went to medical meetings. The month on duty meant that I carried a "beeper" and could be called anytime, days, nights, or weekends, to see patients. I continued to see private patients in the office I shared with Americo in the evenings 2 to 3 days a week. My income from all these activities rose from $13,000 a year in 1964 to $23,000 a year in 1972. Meanwhile, I was buying a house, paying a mortgage, supporting a wife and four daughters, and, beginning in 1972, sending them one at a time to private colleges. Woody helped out by substituting in the Newton public schools and at Perkins School for the Blind.

At dinner I complained about all my problems and this may have discouraged my four girls from ever considering a life in medicine. Between 1963 and 1968, I published only four papers and I was getting criticism from the Public Health Service about the poor productivity on my research grant and my training grant. I was still an associate in medicine at Harvard Medical School and at the Brigham. I asked Dr. Thorn to help me recruit one or two more faculty physicians in gastroenterology but he said that his funds were limited and he first needed to recruit a new chief of hematology and a new chief of cardiology. Americo and I were at the limit of what two people could do. He had five children and his income was as poor as mine. My best fellows, Nuzum, Sarner, Curtis, and

Moritz, had finished their training and I found recruiting new fellows who wanted to do my kind of research was proving difficult. Thus, I began the second five years of my direction of the gastrointestinal division in a state of depression and almost despair.

10

Chief of Gastroenterology

◆

1969–1973

During 1969–1970, I recruited two new fellows, Patricia Ireland and Lennig Chang. When Pat had attended Radcliffe College she was ill much of the time with unexplained abdominal pains. Her doctors thought she had emotional problems. In medical school at the University of Pittsburgh her pains continued, but no cause was found. Finally, when she interned at the Brigham in pathology in 1967–1968, Dr. Perry Culver, a wise senior gastroenterologist at Massachusetts General Hospital, found that she had extensive regional enteritis, an inflammatory disease of the small intestine. She was placed on corticosteroid therapy and her health improved but she paid the price of steroid side effects. I met her in pathology sessions and was pleased to offer her a fellowship. She certainly understood what it was like to suffer from an intestinal disease.

We joined a clinical controlled trial designed by Dr. Harold Conn at Yale, testing whether oral lactulose, a poorly absorbed sugar, reduced the blood ammonia in people with cirrhosis and improved their hepatic encephalopathy. Lactulose was supposed to be a carbon source for the colonic bacteria which would take up ammonia as they multiplied and prevent the ammonia from being absorbed into the blood. Pat agreed to carry out the protocol on patients that we admitted to our clinical research center. These fragile cirrhotic patients were given oral lactulose, which caused diarrhea at the doses planned, or a sweet-tasting placebo sugar containing sorbitol. Clinical tests of hepatic encephalopathy, blood ammonia levels and electro-encephalograms were checked daily. Unfortunately, sorbitol is also a poorly absorbed sugar like lactulose. I counseled Dr. Conn that it might also function like lactulose and would not be a good placebo but he would not change the protocol. The assignments to the treatments were double blind, that is, neither the patient nor the doctors knew which treatment was being given.

Each patient received lactulose or placebo for one week and then the second week the alternate treatment was begun. The pharmacy randomly assigned the patients to start on one treatment or the other and then changed it a week later. After we had processed a number of patients with no differences in their clinical tests or blood ammonias either week of the protocol, I became suspicious that something was wrong. I went to the pharmacist who had been assigned to our study and learned that he had misunderstood the protocol. He sent up lactulose or sorbitol to the ward and alternated the treatments every two days, not every week. The results were therefore meaningless. We were dropped from the study because we failed to follow the protocol and because, in my opinion, sorbitol was equivalent to lactulose. Pat and I were disgusted with the pharmacy because we had lost this work and angry with ourselves because we had not made certain that our pharmacist had read and understood the protocol. Years later, controlled studies showed that lactulose was minimally effective.

Pat decided then that she wanted to review the charts of all the renal transplant patients who developed jaundice, attempting to find out whether their liver injury was due to azathioprine, the drug they were taking to prevent rejection of the transplanted kidney. I warned her that chart reviews might not allow us to tell whether the obstructive hepatitis seen on liver biopsy was due to azathioprine, to one of the many other drugs they were taking or to a hepatitis virus we could not test for. Lennig Chang, our other fellow, had developed a complement fixation test for hepatitis B and he could rule out that disease in the patients she reviewed. After months of work and reviewing masses of data, she concluded that azathioprine was only in a few cases a cause of jaundice of the intrahepatic obstructive type. It was still possible that other viruses and drugs were the cause of these cases. A paper she wrote on this topic was turned down by three journals but was finally published in the *Archives of Internal Medicine.* She was quite discouraged by her attempts to do clinical research and left us after one year to take up a gastroenterology fellowship with Dr. John Fordtran at Southwestern Medical School in Dallas. Pat worked there on small bowel transport but accomplished little, and then left to take another fellowship at the GI division of the New Mexico Medical School in Albuquerque. She again felt that she had accomplished little and after two years went into private practice in Santa Fe, New Mexico. She was successful in her practice but struggled with her regional enteritis. I was told that she died prematurely of its complications. For me this was a tragic loss of a brave, intelligent and caring physician.

Lennig Chang came to us from the University of California–San Francisco Medical School, which he graduated from in 1964. He served his internship and junior residency at the Hartford Hospital in Connecticut and a senior residency at Tufts New England Medical Center. He also served from 1966 to 1968 in Atlanta at the Communicable Disease Center, working on herpes virus in the laboratory. He came to me in 1969 asking to do laboratory research but was not interested in becoming a clinical gastroenterologist. He wanted to work on the newly discovered hepatitis virus called Australia Antigen, later named hepatitis B. Dr. Tom O'Brien, who was now chief of infectious disease, agreed to help him set up a complement fixation assay for hepatitis B. They used the high-titer antibody from an infected hemophiliac patient who got the disease from multiple blood transfusions. Len obtained hepatitis B antigen from our patients with chronic active hepatitis. His complement fixation (CF) method for hepatitis B turned out to be much more sensitive than the previous agar gel diffusion method. While he was setting up this CF assay, we were asked to help study an outbreak of hepatitis in the Holy Cross football team from a water-borne source. Lennig showed that none had hepatitis B. Warren Wacker, Tom O'Brien and Lennig published a paper that showed that the outbreak was due to hepatitis A, the short-incubation form of the disease, spread by fecal contamination of water which the team drank from a faucet near the playing field. Lennig also applied his CF assay to detect hepatitis B in renal transplant patients and in screening blood donors.

Lennig helped me carry out a study comparing the increase in urea cycle enzymes in the liver of rats by casein protein compared with ammonium citrate. In spite of equal increases in urinary urea excretion, the rats fed the protein increased all five urea cycle enzymes while those fed ammonium citrate showed no increases. This result was important since it was previously believed that processing of ammonia nitrogen through the urea cycle in liver led to the adaptive increase in urea cycle enzymes. His previous research in medical school and at Tufts was in immunology, so in 1970 he took a fellowship in rheumatology at Tufts and then another at the Robert Breck Brigham Hospital in 1971. He became an assistant clinical professor of medicine at Tufts University Medical School and then practiced rheumatology at Newton-Wellesley Hospital until his retirement.

Americo and Russell Jeffrey, our former trainee, published a paper in 1969 describing six patients who presented with right upper abdominal pain and markedly elevated levels of serum transaminase enzymes as well as OTC. These patients were misdiagnosed as acute viral hepatitis. Further studies by Dr. Abbruzzese showed that they had acute common bile duct obstruction by migrating gallstones that eventually passed and the enzymes then quickly went back to normal. We jokingly called these cases the "Abbruzzese syndrome."

In 1971, Dr. Thorn told me that Harvard Medical School and Massachusetts Institute of Technology had set up a new experimental pathway through medical school whereby 25 students enrolled at both institutions. They were taught first- and second-year courses by faculty from both schools, stressing the application of basic science to the understanding of medical teachings. Dr. Irving London was made chairman of this Harvard-MIT Program for Health Sciences and began the first-year courses in 1971. Dr. Thorn recommended me to teach the half-semester eight-week course on gastrointestinal pathophysiology in the spring of 1972. I was to be supported by an MIT physics professor and a pathologist from the Beth Israel Hospital. It took me a year to compose the 24 clinical lectures, prepare slides to show during these lectures, plan interesting laboratory exercises and design meaningful tests while doing the rest of my usual teaching and research workload. I asked my former trainee, Martin Sarner, to arrange leave from his duties at University College Hospital in London and give six of the lectures and assist in the laboratory exercises. He enthusiastically agreed and lived with us in our house in Newton for four weeks, finally bringing his wife Nitza and his two young daughters, Shula and Liat, for the last two weeks. While staying with us Nitza became pregnant again with what would be their third daughter, Ilana. The course at MIT went well because we had such bright and eager students and my co-teachers all turned out to be enthusiastic, well prepared, and able to bond with our students. It was a huge challenge for me to master every area of the gastrointestinal tract, liver and pancreas for my lectures and lab exercises. I finally concluded that this experience made me a bona fide consultant in all areas of my specialty. Some of the class members from that group are still friends of mine. The reports on our course were quite positive and even dour Irving London seemed pleased.

My last two fellows were Amer Rayyes and Nazir-uddin Khaja. Recruiting Brigham house staff for our program was no longer successful and applicants from the United States became few in number. I never was certain why this occurred but I believe now that it was because we had only two staff members in the division. Americo and I were obviously overloaded with many responsibilities that prevented us from spending the time needed with our fellows.

Nazir joined us in 1970. He was born in Hyderabad, India, where his father was the prime minister to the Nizam, an incredibly wealthy ruler. After India annexed Hyderabad, Nazir's family moved to Karachi, the capital of Pakistan, where one brother became an admiral in the Pakistan Navy and the other brother the chief pilot of Pakistan Airlines. Nazir chose medicine. He went to medical school in Saudi Arabia and did his house staff training in the United States. He came to our program to learn clinical gastroenterology but he was willing to try clinical research. Nazir compared our serum OTC assay with other liver enzyme tests in 100 patients with different forms of biopsy-proven liver disease. He and I reviewed and graded all of these biopsies and compared them with the enzyme tests. We published an abstract of this work in *Gastroenterology* in 1971 but Nazir never wrote a full paper. He found that the liver-specific OTC assay was not helpful in the differential diagnosis of jaundice but pointed to the liver as the source of the injury when serum enzymes like the transaminases were elevated. Nazir was a consummate gentleman and greatly liked by most of the people at the Brigham. He became a skillful endoscopist under the tutelage of Americo. When he arrived, he brought his new bride, who had been Miss India in the Miss Universe contest. She turned out to be spoiled; unhappy in Boston, she shortly left to go home to her mother. Nazir divorced her and later, when he set up a highly successful practice south of Los Angeles, he met a woman ophthalmologist who joined him in a happy marriage and partnership. He stayed only one year with us. Later, he played a major role in my life by advising me not to take the offer of chief of medicine at the Aga Khan Medical School in Karachi, Pakistan. His reasons all turned out to be accurate and he saved me from an unpleasant experience.

Amer Rayyes joined us in 1971, requesting to do gastrointestinal clinical training primarily. He was born in Damascus, Syria, and went to medical school at the famous American University in Beirut, Lebanon, and did his clinical training there. He was the son of an Arab father and a Syrian Greek mother. He married an Armenian woman whose mother was French. I was astounded that his five-year-old son spoke Arabic, Greek, Armenian and French each to the appropriate grandparent and was also fluent in English. Amer was an excellent clinician and became a skillful endoscopist. He worked in the Brigham alcoholic clinic to supplement his income and became quite interested in alcoholism as a disease and in its complications. When I decided to leave Boston in 1972, he went to New York City and joined the gastrointestinal division at St. Luke's Hospital, managing their alcoholism unit. He moved to California near Los Angeles and carried out a successful gastroenterology and hepatology practice. I lost touch with him after 1974.

Thus in the years 1963 to 1972, I trained ten fellows, of whom eight were eventually in practice and only two remained in academic medicine, namely Tom Nuzum and Martin Sarner. The number of publications by these fellows totaled only ten, a poor yield from the NIH training grant given to us from 1965 to 1972. Finally in 1972, after a site visit from three high-level gastrointestinal experts, my training grant was canceled. This meant that I had no way to pay for new fellows if I could recruit them.

In contrast, the research in my laboratory on urea cycle enzymes began to produce important findings while supported by an NIH grant from 1963 to 1973. My paper in *Biochemistry* in 1968 on the effects of pH on the kinetics of human OTC showed that the true substrate of the reaction was the neutral form of ornithine (the zwitter ion) and that the binding site on the enzyme was a histidine side chain. The liver OTC assay we developed was used worldwide. The serum OTC assay that David Perry and I developed changed the way OTC was measured. The *Science* paper of 1971 with Tom Nuzum proved that primates adapted to the level of dietary protein as did rats. Tom Nuzum's paper in *The Urea Cycle* book (1976) led to the use of our colorimetric microassays of all five urea cycle enzymes throughout the world. Our collaboration with Ingrid Richardson and Armen Tashjian at the Harvard Dental School led to the isolation of the first clonal strain of hepatoma cells which maintained all five urea cycle enzymes in culture (*Journal of Cell Physiology,* 1974).

Meanwhile, I began to collaborate with pediatricians and geneticists in their studies of OTC deficiency in children. We could assay all five enzymes in 10 to 20 mg of liver tissue obtained by needle biopsy and if we had more tissue we could do kinetic studies looking for pH or Km (Michaelis constant) mutants. In 1971, the genetics group at Yale, under Dr. Leon Rosenburg, published the first cases of lethal hyperammonemia in affected males with OTC deficiency. Tom Nuzum and I were coauthors. Dr. Ellen Kang at the Harvard Children's Hospital and I published one of the other early cases of neonatal death in OTC deficient males (*Journal of Pediatrics,* 1973). Finally, in 1973, two papers in the *New England Journal of Medicine* showed the expanded series of lethal deficiency in males from the Yale group and showed in the second paper that this was an X-linked dominant defect. OTC deficiency was the most common genetic defect in the urea cycle and was rarely recognized until these papers were published.

We most importantly proved that all five urea cycle enzymes were induced (increased in activity and amount) in rats by glucagon, a pancreatic hormone, and by cyclic-AMP. We discovered that alanine, a gluconeogenic amino acid, induced the entire cycle as well as an equal nitrogen dose of the protein casein. These findings were presented at meetings of the International Congresses of Gastroenterology in Copenhagen in 1970, in Paris in 1972, and in Madrid in 1978 as well as at meetings of the American Society of Biological Chemists and of the American Gastroenterologic Association. My reputation in this narrow field of the urea cycle was becoming international. Although I was promoted to Assistant Professor of Medicine from Associate in Medicine at Harvard Medical School in 1969, Dr. Thorn explained to me in 1972 that he was retiring and was not allowed to promote me or others to higher faculty positions. This was to be the prerogative of his successor. He also refused to appoint any new members to my division because of lack of money, even though I had interviewed good candidates who wanted to join me.

The new chairman of medicine, announced in 1972, was Dr. Eugene Braunwald, a cardiologist from San Diego, and a man known to be critical and demanding. When he began to visit the Brigham on a part-time basis, I presented a carefully considered plan for enlarging and upgrading the gastrointestinal division. He said that he had consulted with Kurt Isselbacher and other gastrointestinal chiefs about me and was told that I was an excellent performer and only needed support for my division to grow and prosper. As a result he told me that I was his choice to direct the division in the future. He said that he would work with me to enlarge and improve the division. Four months later, at the clinical meetings in Atlantic City, I heard from friends that he was looking for someone to replace me! Faced with this betrayal of trust, I discussed my future with Warren Wacker, Bert Vallee and others of my friends. After a month in Paris at the International Congress of Gastroenterology, agonizing over whether to stay and be downgraded, I decided to look for a new position which would be a step up from being chief of a gastrointestinal division. My friend Tom O'Brien decided to stay at the Brigham even though Dr. Braunwald had chosen a new chief of infectious disease to replace him. After discussing the position of chief of medicine at VA Hospitals with my friend and wife's classmate, Dr. Arthur Sasahara, chief of the medical service at the West Roxbury VA Hospital, I decided this position would be a logical next step up if I could be appointed at a VA Hospital in an academic medical center. After interviews at the University of Connecticut and at Loma Linda, California, where VA positions were offered me, my former student, intern and long time friend, T.K. Li, called me from Indianapolis, where he was now professor of medicine and biochemistry. He told me that the chief of medical service position was open at their VA hospital. He assured me that it was a first-class VA hospital with a total integration of its program with the Indiana University School of Medicine on the same campus. I went to Indianapolis in September of 1972 for an interview with the chairman, Dr. Walter Daly, who seemed to like me and my performance record. He offered me a promotion to full professor (on the volunteer faculty) and the VA offered me a 1500-square-foot laboratory building of my own and the opportunity to apply for VA research funding in addition to my NIH grant. The salary would be twice what I earned at the Brigham and would help me pay for two daughters now in college at Oberlin and Carleton. I accepted the position and was to start in January in 1973, part-time.

Dr. Braunwald looked exceedingly pleased when I told him that I had been offered this position and he advised me to accept it. He said that the Indianapolis VA was an excellent hospital and that he was proud that I would be his first professor. At a later meeting, George Thorn stated that he was proud that I would be his last professor. However, Dr. Braunwald told me that he would not let me leave the Brigham or take any of my laboratory equipment unless I stayed and wrote the grant application for the clinical research center renewal, totaling $12 million, and supervised the site visit in March 1973. The grant was renewed successfully and I left the Brigham on March 30, 1973. Warren Wacker organized a wonderful farewell party for me and Marjorie. My lawyer gave me a new updated will as a present. I left Boston and never received thanks for service to Harvard Medical School from Dean Ebert or thank-you notes from Dr. Braunwald, the chief of surgery, Francis Moore, or the other chiefs of service. The director of the hospital, William Hassan, however, thanked me for a job well done over the years 1953 to 1973. He was counting on Dr. Braunwald to help the Brigham out of its precarious financial position. Dr. Braunwald said as I left, "Tell me George Thorn's secret. How could he vacation in June, July, August and often September each year and still keep the Department of Medicine running well?" I replied that Dr. Thorn had Eugene Eppinger and good senior staff like Lew Dexter and young staff members like Warren Wacker and Dave Ulmer as acting chairmen during those months. He pretended that I never knew about his plans to replace me as chief of gastroenterology. We continued to be civil to each other when we met at meetings. He eventually replaced all of George Thorn's division chiefs with those of his own choosing. The Brigham survived and thrived during his twenty-year tenure and many people came to love and respect him. I felt relieved to be free of his rule.

11

Chief of the VA Medical Service and Professor of Medicine

♦

1973–1981

Before assuming my new position full-time as chief of the medical service at the VA Hospital in Indianapolis, I flew out from Boston to spend one week in January, February, and March 1973 getting my office and research laboratory set up. I hired a new office administrator, Dorothy Bradley. She was a bright and attractive black woman who had climbed from the position of record room clerk to executive secretary in this VA. She knew everyone in the hospital, all the gossip and secrets, so that she could advise me about my interactions with everyone from the director down to the floor cleaners. Medical service had 90 employees and I was their supervisor. The new director, John Peters, was assigned to the Indianapolis VA in 1972 to straighten out its poor administration and relations with the medical school which resulted from the troubled performance of the previous hospital director. John was known in the VA system as one of the top five directors who came out of World War II. He taught me so much about the politics of the VA system and the management of a hospital. My predecessor as chief of medical service, Roy Behnke, had left a year before to become chairman of medicine at the new South Florida School of Medicine in Tampa. He took with him the entire VA renal group, who were caring for the VA Dialysis Program, and the Indiana University Renal Transplant Program, which was based at the VA. He also took the transplant surgeon. Stuart Kleit, chief of the renal division in the Department of Medicine, John Peters, Walter Daly and I made recruiting a new transplant surgeon and new VA renal staff physicians our highest priority. We found a surgeon from the University of Michigan who was trained in liver surgery originally and he accepted. He turned out to be a good but temperamental transplant surgeon. Stuart Kleit assigned one of his recent trainees to take over the VA dialysis unit and he found an experienced renal internist from another school to support the transplant program. We built a new and larger dialysis unit in the main VA hospital on the IU Medical Center Campus and remodeled a ward there for transplant patients. The previous units had been based at our old Cold Springs Road hospital, three miles up the White River. There was no house staff available there for emergencies and the X-ray and laboratory support were inadequate.

I helped Dr. Daly look for a new chief of gastroenterology for University Hospital but none of the people I brought to Indianapolis seemed to please him. So he made Phillip Christiansen the chief, a man who had trained at the Lahey Clinic in Boston in traditional gastroenterology and had been at University Hospital for many years. Because his VA research was not renewed I inherited his space in the research building that became my laboratory.

He also left me three technicians whom I was supposed to support. One tech, named Sharon, was bright but undisciplined and I thought the best of the three. I arranged for her to come to Boston and work in my laboratory for three weeks in February, learning to do urea cycle enzyme assays and the other procedures we used. She returned to Indianapolis and in March set up and practiced all the methods we taught her. I wrote a grant application on new aspects of urea cycle enzyme research using cultured hepatoma (liver tumor) cells we had isolated in Boston. The grant was site visited in February along with the rest of the VA research projects and my project was approved. I now had an NIH grant plus VA funding. I was told that I must take on the other two technicians because they were VA career employees. Catherine Maxey, a 55-year-old black woman, turned out to be smart and experienced and had become bored from doing nothing interesting. She welcomed the challenges of urea cycle work and shortly thereafter I made her my chief technician. The third technician, a 60-year-old man named Bill, had been a sergeant in the Army and knew how to avoid work or pretend to be working. I made him useful by putting him in charge of all the experiments concerning rat diets and feedings. He never learned to do enzyme assays in a dependable way. Thus, when I arrived for full-time duty on April 1, 1973, my lab was up and running and experiments were being done.

The Associate Chief of Staff for Research was Dr. Norman Bell, a prominent endocrinology investigator. He was the first person at the VA to befriend me, asking me to dinner, where I met his wife, Ledlie, and his children. He helped me write my VA research grant and get to know staff members at the VA hospital.

When I arrived as a full-time employee on April Fool's Day, I left behind my wife and children to sell our house in Newton and to move our household goods into the 1960-vintage house on a creek which Woody found during a visit in February. I had been advised to move the two youngest girls, Amy (13) and Emily (7), in May so that they could attend the schools in Washington Township and get to know classmates and teachers. Jennifer stayed in Newton during the month of May with friends and finished high school and then Woody and I went back in June for her graduation from Newton South High School. Martha was finishing her first year at Oberlin College. Jennifer had been admitted to Carleton College for the fall of 1973. She and Martha Sue never really accepted the house in Indianapolis as their new home. Amy and Emily did accept the move and made new friends and eventually were happy in their new schools. Indianapolis had been Woody's birthplace and home through high school. Her father, a 40-year teacher of German and Spanish at Arsenal Technical High School, had died in 1968. Her stepmother, Flora, retired as a nurse from the Marion County Tuberculosis Association and lived in the family home, first with boarders and then alone. Flora hosted me when I came to work at the VA for one week a month the first three months of 1973. Flora then became the grandmother figure Amy and Emily needed in Indianapolis. Woody had other family friends, especially Iris Myers, who cared for her at age 7 to 9 after her mother died of leukemia. We joined a small Presbyterian church nearby, where we found new friends. Our new home was close to downtown and to Butler University. We subscribed to the Indianapolis Symphony Orchestra concerts and also attended the many theater and music group performances in Indianapolis. T.K. Li and his wife Susan invited us to dinner on a number of occasions. Amy and Emily became friends with their daughters Jennifer and Karen. Indianapolis turned out to be a good place for us to live.

My first month at the VA, I assigned myself as one of the attending physicians on a ward to establish my clinical credentials. The resident, two interns and four students were eager to test out this new chief of medicine. I fear that I showed off, displaying my internal medicine knowledge and my diagnostic skills. The chief of the gastroenterology section at the VA was a pleasant man who had struggled unsuccessfully to do laboratory research and had lost his VA research grant. When we worked together in the gastroenterology clinic, we differed on the care of some diseases. He had never learned to do endoscopy so we had to bring a person over from the University Hospital to do our cases or I would have to substitute in an emergency. I insisted that he learn upper (gastroduodenal) and lower (colonic) endoscopy and he became quite skilled at it. By the end of 1973, he told me that he was leaving the VA and going into private practice at one of the large private hospitals. There he was successful and expressed gratitude to me for helping him change his career.

I found his replacement in a man named Lawrence Lumeng, who was finishing his third year of VA sponsored research training. Larry attended Indiana University School of Medicine, interned at the University of Chicago Hospitals and returned to our medical center for his second and third years of training. He obtained a master's degree in the biochemistry department with Professor Jack Davis, an expert in mitochondrial function. Larry then went into the U.S. Army and was assigned to Walter Reed Army Hospital, where he met T.K. Li, who was also assigned there. They developed an alcohol-preferring strain of rats by selective breeding. They brought this unique animal model with them to Indianapolis when T.K. was appointed professor of medicine and biochemistry by John Hickam, then chairman of medicine. Larry entered the VA research fellowship program and continued to work with Dr. Li. Once I met Larry, I knew we were soul mates. We were both trained in biochemistry and were doing biochemistry research. We were interested mainly in liver disease and not interested in doing endoscopy. I appointed him as chief of GI at the VA and we shared the weekly gastroenterology-liver clinic duties for the next twenty years. He and T.K. Li continued to do studies together using the alcohol-preferring rats.

The Dean of Indiana University School of Medicine when I was hired in 1973 was Dr. Glen Irwin. He warmly welcomed me and told me that they were quite pleased to find a person of my caliber to take over the medical service at the VA. He approved my promotion from assistant professor at Harvard to full professor at IU School of Medicine. T.K. Li explained to him and Walter Daly that the Harvard title "Associate in Medicine" was equivalent to assistant professor in other schools. I did not at first realize that the appointment was to the volunteer faculty, not the full-time faculty, a situation in which all our full-time VA doctors found themselves. I was not listed in the Indiana University Faculty Handbook and when I asked about it, they said that only faculty receiving Indiana University salary were considered true members of the University. My entire salary was paid by the VA, even though I served on many medical school committees and taught students and house staff. I was elected to three terms on the faculty promotions and tenure committee by my fellow faculty members. My VA salary initially was $50,000, a huge jump up from my Brigham income. Within a few years, the salaries of full professors at the IU School of Medicine climbed to a $100,000 per year. I asked Dr. Daly whether he would not try to bring me and my VA doctors closer to the salaries of those of the same rank at the University

Hospital. For two years, he added the supplement of $2,000 to my salary and then stopped it, pleading inability to generate enough funds from the Department of Medicine to do more. From then on to retirement, I requested a supplement from each of the two new departmental chairmen and all denied my requests. A study done in the VA system showed that in 22 of 25 large academic VA hospitals, the chief of medical service was supplemented by the medical school or the department of medicine. I regretted that I did not make this a part of my recruitment agreement when I first came to Indiana.

My second Dean was Steven Beering, a German refugee and former U.S. Air Force colonel who came to Indiana University to set up the statewide educational system. In this system, the first and often the second years of medical school were offered at universities around the state, such as Indiana University, Notre Dame, Purdue, Ball State, Indiana State and others. All students finished their last two years in Indianapolis for their clinical training. The class grew to 290, the largest in the nation. This program prevented the Indiana legislature from setting up four-year medical schools all over the state. This proliferation occurred in Illinois and caused a severe problem maintaining high and equal standards at these small schools. I once asked Steve if he would create a separate clinical track for medical school professors who did not do research or publish and did mostly clinical practice which supported the various departments and subsidized the basic science departments. He said "You do research, obtain grants, publish papers and still do a heavy load of patient care, teaching and committee work. Why do you want to cheapen our full-time professorships by creating a clinical nonacademic track?" He never did so during his tenure. When he left to become president of Purdue University in 1983, Dr. Walter Daly was chosen as dean and established this clinical track. It had become obvious in our school and medical schools across the country that they were not financially viable unless they had a cadre of "worker bees" who did clinical practice and contributed a large part of their income to their departmental chairman and dean.

At the Brigham, my old partner Americo Abbruzzese was now part of a gastrointestinal division of eight people headed by Dr. Jerry Trier. Dr. Braunwald made a rule that all Department of Medicine income must go to his office and then he negotiated how much salary each faculty member was paid. Americo generated $150,000 from his heavy endoscopy and clinic care schedules, but he was paid only $64,000 by Dr. Braunwald. The balance was used to pay the researchers who did not generate a salary from their grants and from their sparse clinical duties. When I visited Americo and he told me this tale at dinner, I strongly advised him to leave the Brigham and go into private practice on the North Shore of Boston, where he lived, and stop being exploited by Dr. Braunwald and Dr. Jerry Trier. He had six children by now, with four of them in college. He followed my advice and soon was seeing patients in a number of North Shore hospitals. He became highly respected and well-to-do and was able to educate his children and save for retirement. Departmental chairman all over the United States adopted Braunwald's method of financing their departments. Walter Daly never did this when he was chairman but levied a chairman's tax on each division and the dean also levied a tax on each department.

Shortly after I arrived at the VA, it became apparent to me that as chief of the medical service, I could not spend more than a few minutes with each technician, each morning and late afternoon. T.K. Li advised me that I should hire a person with a PhD to supervise my laboratory and research. He had in mind a woman in the Department of Biochemistry whose mentor was leaving. Renee Lin was raised in Taiwan, did her college work there and then luckily was accepted at the University of Wisconsin Department of Biochemistry with a famous professor with whom she obtained her PhD. Her thesis concerned mitochondrial functions. Her husband, a statistician, came to Indianapolis to work for Eli Lilly Company. In spite of her excellent training, she could only find a super-technician's job in the Department of Biochemistry at our medical school. I changed my grants so that I could offer her a good salary and obtained for her an appointment as lecturer in medicine and biochemistry. She eagerly accepted and quickly made herself an expert in urea cycle biochemistry and learned to do cell culture.

Our hepatoma cell line did not respond to hormonal stimuli. At a meeting in Chicago, I heard of a method for isolating and maintaining liver cells on plastic dishes. Renee and I tried this and she improved the method by coating the plates with collagen and using a serum-free growth medium, which kept the cells alive for a week with a minimal loss of urea cycle enzyme activities. The five enzymes all increased in activity when exposed to glucagon or cyclic AMP. Thus, we had a cell culture system in which to study enzyme induction. We published this method in *Biochemical Biophysical Research Communications* in 1975. Many other laboratories used it or modified it for their own purposes.

Renee wanted to establish a career and reputation separate from mine, hoping to be promoted to Assistant Professor at the Medical School. Using her cultured liver cell system, she discovered that the cells would maintain the activity of HMGCoA reductase, the key enzyme in cholesterol synthesis. This enzyme, the one inhibited by the "statin drugs" to lower human cholesterol levels, she found was induced by a corticosteroid. Her paper in *Federation of European Biochemical Societies Letters* in 1977 began her independent research career. Meanwhile, I published a major paper in the *Journal of Biological Chemistry*, the premiere journal in the field, about the induction of the urea cycle by glucagon.

After the *New England Journal* papers on OTC deficiency, I received many telephone calls from pediatricians and geneticists requesting help studying children and adults with urea cycle enzyme deficiencies. We collaborated by doing liver enzyme assays and kinetic studies if adequate liver tissue was available from children with various urea cycle deficiencies. I was listed as a coauthor when papers were published about carbamyl phosphate synthetase (CPS), ornithine transcarbamylase, argininosuccinate lyase, and arginase deficiencies.

Before we left Boston, I had learned about a new syndrome in children in which, after various viral infections, they developed nausea, severe vomiting, confusion, then coma and often died of brain swelling due to high blood ammonia levels. This syndrome was first described by R.D.K. Reye, a pediatrician in Santiago, Chile, and colleagues in the *Lancet* journal in 1963. I learned from my pediatric collaborator, Ellen Kang, that some of these children had low to absent serum citrulline levels. This suggested a defect in either CPS or OTC, the mitochondrial enzymes of the urea cycle. I was able to obtain liver tissue from eight cases at Boston Children's Hospital and Riley Hospital for Children in Indianapolis and found as suspected OTC activities below normal in seven out of eight and CPS levels low in two of eight. The other urea cycle enzymes in the cytoplasm were normal. The residual OTC activity had normal pH optimums and binding constants for the substrates (K_ms). So we concluded that there was a deficiency in a normal OTC enzyme, not a genetic defect. We collaborated with a neurologist at Massachusetts General Hospital, who measured urinary urea and nitrogen in two patients. The nitrogen excretion was massive, suggesting severe tissue breakdown, but only 20 to 40% of the urine nitrogen had been converted into urea. Normally 80 to 90% of urinary nitrogen is in the form of urea. We concluded that Reye's syndrome was associated with severe mitochondrial damage in the liver. Later, mitochondrial injury in brain and muscle was proven. The paper by Snodgrass and DeLong in the *New England Journal* (1976) was paired with another paper showing the same CPS and OTC enzyme defects.

The epidemic of Reye's syndrome in the United States lasted from 1965 to 1980 and then resolved. Epidemiological evidence suggested that aspirin ingestion during the viral illness might trigger Reye's syndrome. Aspirin was given warning labels by the Food and Drug Administration and families were urged to avoid aspirin when their child had a viral illness. This abolishing of aspirin use was given credit for the near disappearance of Reye's syndrome. However, some of our cases had no history of aspirin ingestion and no aspirin in their blood.

Eventually, it turned out that most cases of Reye's syndrome were due to genetic defects in mitochondrial metabolism of various sorts. The true Reye's syndrome as an entity is now rarely seen and a connection between the viral illness and the onset of the syndrome has never been explained. A number of cases were called Reye's syndrome but turned out to be mild OTC deficiency unmasked by the negative nitrogen balance of their febrile illness, a well-known precipitating cause of coma in such children. My reputation in the world of liver disease was elevated by the work on Reye's syndrome and I was asked to give lectures on it and urea cycle deficiencies at a number of meetings. The highlight was being asked to give a talk at the plenary session of the Digestive Disease Week meetings in San Antonio, Texas, in 1975. I was later asked to give the lecture on urea cycle enzyme deficiencies at a symposium in 1980, which was published in the *Journal of Pediatrics* in 1981.

Tom Nuzum asked me to lecture on pancreatic disease at the University of Kentucky School of Medicine in their second-year course on the biology of disease each spring from 1973 to 1977. This gave me a chance to stay with Tom and his wife Jean, and get to know their daughter Caroline and son Henry. I visited hospitals around Indiana as part of the visiting professor program, talking about pancreatic and biliary tract diseases. These lectures allowed me to keep up with the graduates of our internal medicine programs who were now practicing in various cities.

One of the most satisfying aspects of being chief of the medical service at the VA was that I could choose the chief residents who spent the entire academic year with me. I tried to teach them as much as I knew about internal medicine, teaching, leadership of residents and students, the ethics of medicine and the politics of medicine. They became the sons in medicine I never had because none of my daughters or sons-in-law chose a medical career. These men were an outstanding group, better in my opinion than the chief residents chosen at the University Hospital and at the county hospital (Wishard Hospital). My first chief resident, Horace "Bud" Hickman, in 1973–1974, trained in cardiology and became the leader in cardiology at St. Francis Hospital on the south side of Indianapolis. L. Samuel Wann, 1974–1975, also trained in cardiology and in the new cardiac ultrasound methods. He was made an assistant professor at the University of Wisconsin at Milwaukee School of Medicine. Samuel Milligan trained in renal medicine and ended up running the dialysis unit and renal division in a large hospital in South Bend, Indiana. Gerald Braverman practiced internal medicine at St. Francis Hospital and became a leader in their hospital. Robert Daly trained in pulmonary medicine and went to St. Francis to supervise their intensive care unit. He "moonlighted" at night to gain extra money in their intensive care unit while still serving as my chief resident. One night our chairman, Walter Daly, received a call asking him to come immediately to St. Francis to help with a patient in pulmonary failure. Walter guessed that they were looking for Robert Daly. He called Bob the next day and told him they should never call Walter Daly by mistake again. William Hyde went to Princeton, Illinois, near his hometown to practice internal medicine and to serve as director of medical education. Robert Hoerr wanted to do research in nutrition. I was able to obtain a fellowship for him at the Nutrition Research Unit at Massachusetts Institute of Technology in Boston. When Bob was chief resident, we were assigned a new hospital director who was not smart or sensible. Moreover, "Mac" was stubborn and would not listen to advice. In order to fill our medical wards and thereby increase reimbursement from the VA, he told the nurses to place beds in the halls, where there was no oxygen or other support systems. There were not enough nurses on these wards to care for the extra patients. Bob called me in the middle of the night to say that the director had ordered this and beds were being placed in the halls at that moment. I drove to the hospital and Bob and I took the beds out of halls and down the elevators to the basement and ordered the nurses and night administrative staff to disobey the director's orders. The next morning, I faced down "Mac" and convinced him not to do this again. I explained to him that he was not a doctor and should not issue orders which impaired patient care. Rex Flygt, my next chief resident, went into practice in Baraboo, Wisconsin. David Buchner had majored in experimental psychology at Harvard College and wanted to find a career where he could use his knowledge. I encouraged him to apply for a Robert Wood Johnson fellowship in epidemiology at the University of Washington in Seattle. Dave was accepted and did so well that they eventually made him a professor of medicine and public health; he excelled in teaching and in the new area of patient care research. I consider these men as one of the most satisfying products of my career in academic medicine. I had offered the position to three of the outstanding women coming through our program but up to 1982 none accepted because they thought the culture at the VA would not welcome a female chief resident.

My laboratory technicians kept leaving for better-paying jobs and more stable positions, just as they did in Boston. I always encouraged them to pursue this upward mobility. Two in Boston made it to medical school and are practicing physicians. After Sharon left to follow her husband to Florida, I hired a husband and wife who had earned master's degrees in biochemistry in India. They were marvelous people and I felt sorry to see them to go to Baylor University Medical

School in Houston, Texas, where they were given positions with long-term appointments. I visited them once and was treated royally as they put on a dinner for me with all their friends. This technician turnover meant that I had to train new people in all the complex methods of our lab over and over. It took three to four months before I could rely on them to work alone on their own projects. One woman left after three months for another job she had actually applied for before I even hired her.

I used the position of dishwasher in our laboratory as a way to help out people not likely to be hired by others. To do chemically clean washing of our glassware was essential for enzyme assays and required careful but tedious effort. A mildly retarded woman learned the job, her first ever, but then became pregnant by someone in her family and had to leave. A man with quite severe cerebral palsy learned to do the job but then became obsessed with one of my new female technicians. He accosted her in the laboratory, called her by phone constantly and would not stop even after I discussed this with him. Finally, I let him go and she left for a better job with Dow Chemical Company. Catherine Maxey supervised these dishwashers for twenty years and helped me continue the policy of hiring minorities and disabled people in spite of some disappointing experiences.

In 1980, I learned that Dr. Donald Doolittle at the veterinary school in Purdue had discovered a new mutant mouse which had a genetic deficiency of ornithine transcarbamylase or OTC. He called these sparse fur (spf) mice because the affected males were born hairless and then he added the superscript "ash" (abnormal skin and hair) to the spf to distinguish them from a sparse fur mouse discovered at Oak Ridge Laboratory in Tennessee. I hired a woman with training in animal care and breeding and, with Dr. Doolittle's help, set up a breeding colony of the spf^{ash} mice in our VA animal quarters. We discovered that the males had about 10% of normal mouse liver OTC levels and that the enzymes had normal pH optimums and substrate binding constants. The males were still able to breed with females so we were able to produce a homozygous mutant female with 10% of OTC activity. The female carriers had OTC activities in their livers ranging from 10 to 80% of normal, averaging 50%. This is because females are X-chromosome mosaics. Their liver cells are made up randomly of genes containing normal or, in this case, abnormal X-chromosomes. We planned to use these mice as animal models of mild OTC deficiency and test out enzyme induction by hormones or by certain amino acids.

Bill was given a project to tube-feed individual amino acids to rats over 48 hours. This was to follow up on our Boston observation that the amino acid alanine would induce all five urea cycle enzymes as well as the protein, casein, when given in equal nitrogen-containing doses. Bill gave maximally tolerated doses of 20 different amino acids and found that only four of them induced all five urea cycle enzymes. The first two, alanine and glycine, are gluconeogenic amino acids. This means that they are degraded to form glucose. Cysteine is a sulfur-containing amino acid which is also degraded to glucose. Methionine is a sulfur-containing amino acid which is essential in the diet. It cannot be made from other amino acids as are alanine, glycine and cysteine. Other amino acids we tested induced none or only one or two enzymes. A combination of alanine, methionine and glycine in a standard nitrogen-containing dose increased all five enzymes to a greater extent than did an equal nitrogen dose of casein protein. The keto acids of alanine or methionine, which have the alpha-amino group removed, did not induce so it was obvious that intact amino acids were necessary. These findings were surprising and important and were published in the *Journal of Nutrition* in 1981 in an article entitled "Induction of Urea Cycle Enzymes of Rat Liver by Amino Acids" by Snodgrass and Lin. I was asked to be a visiting professor in the Department of Biochemistry at North Carolina State University primarily to discuss these amino acid inductions of the urea cycle enzymes.

One of the great pleasures of my faculty position was the chance to advise medical students about their internship choices. When third-year students made ward rounds with me as their attending physician several asked me to be their intern advisor. One man was expected to graduate near the top of his class and told me that he wanted to train outside Indiana, where he had had all of his education. I gave him a list of the top internal medicine programs in the U.S. and he was fortunate to be chosen by the Department of Medicine at the Texas-Southwestern Medical School, whose chairman was Donald Seldin, a famous and demanding figure in American medicine. Our Indiana man did so well that Dr. Seldin chose him to be his chief resident. Our chairman, Dr. Walter Daly, was unhappy with me that I sent him away from our internal medicine program because he wanted our best medical students to stay at home. A few years later another top student asked me to help him obtain an internship in Boston. I was able to help him be chosen in internal medicine at the Brigham and Women's Hospital (the successor to the Peter Bent Brigham). He did so well there that the house staff supervisor told me that "he was a legend in his own time." He went on to be a professor of medicine and hematology in Louisiana. Again Dr. Daly criticized me for sending him away, stating that such students never return to Indiana. I understood that this was often true but I was proud that our good students could excel at the best hospitals in the country.

One of my advisees ended up near the bottom of his class and was not matched at any of the twelve emergency medicine programs to which he applied. Our dean of students told me that it was my job to call around the country and find him some type of internship. Finally a friend and faculty member at the University of Illinois School of Medicine in Champaign-Urbana agreed to take him into their internal medicine program. My student did not want to work as hard as internal medicine interns were expected to perform and only grudgingly accepted the position. I made him promise to do his best for his own sake, for our school's sake and for the sake of the Illinois program. To my surprise and pleasure he became one of their best interns and obtained a residency in a good emergency medicine program in Arizona.

I enjoyed caring for our veteran patients in the gastrointestinal/liver clinic and as an attending physician on our medical wards. They were usually seriously ill and afflicted with diseases of many organs. Diagnosing and treating these diseases required all the knowledge and skill I could muster. Our medical school interns, residents and students all rotated through the VA hospital and found the care of patients there as challenging as did I and my staff physicians. Almost all of these trainees enjoyed working with the veterans, who liked their young doctors and accepted them as well-motivated caregivers. My credo was that our veteran patients should receive care as good as that available at the other hospitals in our medical center. Making this come true was a never-ending battle as VA funding rose and fell, staff physicians came and went, administrators proved good or bad, nursing staffing became limiting and support from the medical school departments waxed and waned. Our program of continual quality improvement on the medical service served as the model for the other hospital services. During my last ten years our regional director in Ann Arbor, Michigan, and the VA Central Office in Washington, D.C., designated the Richard L. Roudebush VA Medical Center in Indianapolis as one of the "flagship" hospitals in the VA system.

When I joined the VA, various people told me that it was impossible to fire a civil service employee for incompetence. I was soon put to the test. A technician worked for me in our hematology-oncology clinic. Her job was to do white blood cell and platelet counts on patients in the clinic who were receiving chemotherapy or trying to survive with a disease that impaired their bone marrow function. The results of her counts needed to be accurate and available quickly because these numbers were used to decide about chemotherapy or platelet transfusions. The chief of my hematology section told me that her count results were always checked later in the main hematology lab, where machines counted the white cells and platelets and low counts were also checked by manual methods. These results were obtained late in the day so they could not be used to direct treatment in the clinic. Our technician's results were frequently far off from those of the main lab. She was counseled by her clinic director and by me on numerous occasions to be more careful and she was checked on her counting techniques. When no improvement occurred over three months, I consulted our human resources director about how to discharge her for inability to perform her assigned tasks. They said it would take six months of documented counseling, written warnings and collection of results compared with those of the main laboratory. When I did all this and submitted the results to the civil service commission in Washington, D.C., they said I had to do it all over again. Monitoring her results alone was prejudicial since I did not monitor the results of all other technicians on my service compared to a standard laboratory. So I began a monitoring program for every technician on my service. The hematology technician still could not come up with accurate results and we had to have another technician come to the clinic and repeat her counts. Finally, after six months more, I resubmitted the request to separate her from her job at this hospital and they said that they would accept our request. The woman heard about this ruling and quickly submitted her resignation so that being fired would not be on her record. A month later, I received a call from the director of the hematology laboratory in a local hospital asking for a recommendation for this woman who was applying for a similar job at their place. The VA told me that I could only say that she resigned on such a date and could not mention her inability to do simple blood counts. The tenacity that I showed in going through the process of discharging an employee who was a danger to good patient care was noted by my other medical service employees. I never had to go through another such process because my people knew that I expected good to excellent job performance and I would spend whatever time and effort it took to get rid of people who could not do their jobs correctly.

A problem arose with the two doctors who were in charge of my pulmonary ward. The chief of our pulmonary section was a poor administrator and never required our nine pulmonary technicians to cover the wards 24 hours a day. We had only one technician on the night shift covering the intensive care unit (ICU) and four wards. This doctor refused to change their work assignments because they threatened him with a complaint to the employee's union. I took over supervision of the pulmonary section from him and hired a strong-minded, competent woman as chief technician. I rewrote the work schedules so all technicians worked an equal number of day, evening and night shifts covering the ICU and wards 24 hours per day. The union called a job action against me but I won the argument on the basis that patient care came first, not the convenience of the technicians. I convinced the director to hire five more technicians to improve this new staffing program.

The assistant chief of the pulmonary section was a man who had problems relating to the house staff. He got into shouting matches with residents who would not do things exactly his way. His treatment rules were arbitrary and not always the only way to do things. Walter Daly heard from me and from some of the residents how difficult this man could be. Walter served as attending physician on our pulmonary ward one month and observed the problems. He decided that the pulmonary ward, containing only lung cancer cases and patients with chronic obstructive pulmonary disease, was not a good learning experience for the residents. Then we agreed to remove this physician from the Indiana University faculty, where he had no tenure. However, I found out that he had tenure in the VA system. Fortunately, there was an opening for a pulmonary physician at the VA hospital in Danville, Illinois, and we transferred him there. I appointed Ian Dowdeswell, a British-trained pulmonologist, as the chief of the pulmonary section. We closed the pulmonary ward and made it a general medical ward. The former chief of the section thanked me for relieving him of administrative burdens he disliked and freeing him to do clinical research, which he loved. The doctor at Danville was a big success there and was made chief of their medical services. We served together on VA committees and he thanked me for opening up his new career. This experience in the pulmonary section served as a warning to those doctors in my other specialty sections that I expected their clinics and sections to run well, expected them to teach residents and students well and to keep their employees happy and hard-working. Because of the VA research program, my ability to shelter research time for young faculty and the option to work part-time at other hospitals on the campus, I soon recruited a group of the best young academic physicians on the faculty to work at the VA. Their presence improved our patient care and our teaching as well as our research.

During this period, from 1973 to 1981, my family had been flourishing. Martha graduated from Oberlin College in 1976, after being inducted into their chapter of Phi Beta Kappa. She majored in Russian and German and became fluent in both. She also studied piano at the Oberlin Conservatory. In her junior year she won study abroad positions in Heidelberg University in Germany for a semester and at Leningrad University in the Soviet Union for a semester. Her gymnastic training in high school and college made it possible for her to be a member of the gymnastic team in Leningrad. Then she returned to graduate from Oberlin and later entered graduate school in Slavic studies at Indiana University, obtaining a master's degree and editing their newsletter. She then won a scholarship to the Free University of Berlin to study East German politics and hopefully to finish a PhD. However, she spent the year looking for jobs in Europe and ended up in Munich working for Radio Liberty, where she translated Russian articles and reports into English and edited their bulletin.

Jennifer graduated from Carleton College in Minnesota in 1977, also being elected to Phi Beta Kappa. She majored in English and in her senior year was chosen as an intern at Viking Press in New York City to learn about the publishing business. In college, she played her cello in the orchestra and in a string quartet, bought a new cello from a local instrument dealer and took lessons from a member of the Minnesota Orchestra. She was chosen to serve as one of the student representatives on the search committee for a new president of Carleton College. After her internship, Viking offered her a full-time job and she worked her way up to be a young acquisition editor in the New York City publishing business. She played her cello in the orchestra at the 92nd Street YMHA. I visited her regularly and she taught me about New York City as she moved from one part of the city to another.

Amy also chose to go to Carleton College, entering in 1977 and majoring in geology and chemistry. She helped integrate the boys' hockey team and worked on the grounds crew. She was chosen to spend a term in a program of underwater biology on Catalina Island and at Monterey, California. After a job in the Forest Service studying the recovery from the volcanic eruption at Mt. St. Helens, she came to Boston and found work in laboratories at Harvard University. First she was a lab assistant in college chemistry, then a lab technician in the Hydrology Laboratory and finally the analytic chemist in the conservation lab at the Fogg Art Museum for ten years. When the position was eliminated, she obtained a master's degree in the history of science at Harvard. Now she is pursuing her interest in sailing ships and in museum work.

During her senior year in high school Amy had a German "sister" living with us. She was an exchange student of the American Field Service from Kassel, Germany, named Sabine Wunsch. Sabine had a great experience in an American high school, so different from the classical Gymnasium in Kassel where her father was headmaster. She played flute in the marching band and enjoyed her four new Snodgrass sisters. She returned home to finish the Gymnasium, was admitted to medical school in Göttingen and graduated into an internship in Hildesheim, where the medical student she married also trained. She and her father and mother became close friends with all of us and we visited in each others' homes.

Emily did well in the Washington Township school system. She took part in gymnastics, ballet and the concert and marching bands, playing the flute. Marjorie worked one year as a secretary in the Inter-Church center and then returned to college at Butler University to get her teacher's certificate for teaching the blind, the visually handicapped and the mildly mentally impaired. She also received a master's degree in education, completing what she began in 1950 at the Harvard School of Education. Then she taught at the Indiana School for the Blind for two years and in 1979 became the only certified teacher of the visually handicapped in the Indianapolis Public Schools. Her class of junior high students included multiply handicapped as well as visually impaired students. Her program was moved from school to school every year for no apparent reason and she had to adjust to good and bad school principals as well as to difficult and arbitrary administrators in the Indianapolis Public School system. With Emily a junior in high school, I began to plan for a sabbatical leave in 1981.

12

Sabbatical Leave

◆

1982

I asked Walter Daly, my chairman of medicine, if he would approve a sabbatical leave for me in 1982. My tenure at Indiana University School of Medicine was then eight years. He agreed if I could find someone to replace me as chief of the medical service at the VA while I was gone. Dean Steven Beering also approved, with the proviso that my replacement would serve on my various medical school committees. The new director at the VA was agreeable but pointed out that I needed permission from VA Central Office in Washington, D.C., and only would be given six months' leave at full salary. The research service in VA Central Office said that they would need to approve the place I chose to work and study and that I should write a grant application to do research in my funded area of urea cycle studies. Therefore I looked for a laboratory where I could do research which would expand my capabilities and scope in the urea cycle area. After careful consideration and consulting various colleagues in Europe, I chose the Metabolic Research Laboratory in Oxford, England, hoping that the director, Sir Hans Krebs, would agree to make me a visiting scientist for six months. I was slightly acquainted with Professor Krebs from talking with him at meetings and he knew that I worked on the urea cycle. He had discovered the urea/ornithine cycle as a young man in Freiburg, Germany, in 1932. Because he had Jewish parents, the Nazis forced him out and he made his way to Cambridge University in England. When no permanent appointment was offered there or at Oxford, he became professor of pharmacology in Sheffield University, then a second-level institution. He set up his laboratory and recruited technicians and one PhD candidate to continue the metabolic studies in liver slices using the Warburg manometric methods he was taught in Otto Warburg's lab. In 1936, J. A. Johnson and Krebs published a report that showed another cycle was present in liver mitochondria. This cycle in nine steps accomplished the breakdown of pyruvic acid, the end product of glucose degradation in the cytoplasm, to generate hydrogens which fed into the electron transport chain and produced ATP. The carrier molecule in this cycle was oxaloacetic acid. It was regenerated with each turn of the cycle and combined with another pyruvic acid to form citric acid. This Krebs or citric acid cycle won him the Nobel Prize in physiology and medicine in 1953 and appointment as head of biochemistry at Oxford University. He retired at age 65 and now, almost 80, was still productive in his own laboratory, the Metabolic Research Laboratory at the Radcliffe Infirmary in Oxford. When I requested to work on some aspect of the urea cycle, he explained that only one person, Patricia Lund, was still working in that area. If I agreed to work with her and supplied my own salary and supplies, he would welcome me for six months. So Pat Lund and I consulted and wrote a proposal to study human liver glutaminase, the enzyme which splits glutamine into glutamic acid and ammonia. The ammonia then feeds into the urea cycle. I sent this research proposal to Research Service at VA Central Office and my six-month sabbatical was approved. I then set out to arrange coverage for my laboratory and the medical service. Renee Lin was completely competent to supervise my laboratory. We planned six months of experiments in general and agreed that she would consult with me weekly by telephone about progress and problems. My clinical replacement was to be my assistant chief of medical service, Ian Dowdeswell. He was raised in Kenya, the son of a microbiologist. He was sent to England for public schooling. He then trained in medicine at St. Thomas's Hospital medical school in London and did his residency training in Capetown, South Africa. He later did postgraduate work at the Brompton Hospital in London on pulmonary diseases. Rhodesia, where he practiced and lived with his wife, son and two girls, became Zimbabwe after a civil war. It then was governed by a radical President Mugabe who subsequently drove white settlers off their farms and made Harare, the capital, unsafe and a poor place to practice medicine. So Ian came to Indianapolis to interview for a position on our faculty. I met and liked him and told him that I would make him chief of the VA pulmonary section once he obtained his green card. He worked at the Wishard (County) Hospital for one year and then was accepted at the VA when he became a legal resident. I found him to be strong in clinical care, but not much interested in research. He became the director and main staff person of our intensive care unit. I trusted him to keep the service running well. He had a warm relationship with my chief resident, Jack Coggeshall.

    I talked to Hans Krebs about our plans in September and everything looked ready to go for February 1982. In November, Derek Williamson, a senior member in Krebs's lab, visited Indianapolis and asked to talk to me. He said that the "Prof," as they called him, had metastatic melanoma and was not expected to live long. A mole on his back had begun to grow in the summer and by September when it was removed it had already spread to his liver and lungs. He was finishing his autobiography. Derek asked if I still wished to come in February, even if Professor Krebs were not there. My dream had been to work with him and learn the secrets of how he did research and stayed productive even at the age of 80. So much effort had gone into preparing for this sabbatical that I did not want to back out now. So I told Derek and Pat Lund that I was coming as planned. Hans Krebs died in December 1981, having seen the first copy of his autobiography.

On February 1, 1982, my wife, Marjorie, daughter Emily and I flew to London where we were met by my former fellow Martin Sarner. He had rented a van and drove us and our copious luggage to Oxford. Pat Lund had found us a splendid flat on the near north side of Oxford, across from the famous Dragon School and within walking distance of the laboratory in Radcliffe Infirmary. Our landlady, Lady Patricia Freeman, had inherited a large house from her husband as well as his title. She was a former dancer who met her husband during World War II at a serviceman's club. She lived on the first floor. Our flat was on the second and third floors; off to the side, an elderly couple lived in a flat on the second floor. We became good friends with Patricia and she introduced Marjorie, no longer called Woody in Oxford, to the Newcomers Club. There she met Oxford University wives and wives of foreign visitors. She went hiking once a week with the "Ramblers" group and attended special functions. Pat Lund arranged for me to become a member of the common room at Green College, the newly created home for the medical students at Oxford. It was adjacent to Radcliffe Infirmary. We often ate lunch there and regularly attended the formal Thursday night dinners in the famous "Tower of the Winds," the building around which the college was built. Sir Richard Doll was president of Green College and he and his wife welcomed us warmly. Doll was the epidemiologist who first reported that smoking caused lung cancer and other cancers in his famous 1952 paper about smoking and cancer in British physicians.

Pat took me to the Metabolic Research Laboratory (MRL) and introduced me to all the staff. This famous laboratory was merely a bridge between two buildings with a driveway beneath us. Everyone worked in one large room at benches serving both for research and writing desks. A cubbyhole on one side had been Professor Krebs's office, with no door, From there he kept an eye on everyone in the room. A separate room was for instruments and another room for the library and his secretary, Madge. I was assigned a bench and a small desk. Contrary to most visiting professors at the MRL, I insisted on doing my own experiments and did not ask for a technician to help. David, the technician across the bench from me, was amazed because he always was assigned to help visiting professors. The dishwasher, an elderly lady, was surprised when I came in at 8 a.m. Everyone else showed up at 9 a.m. and worked diligently under the supervision of the senior staff, Pat Lund, Derek Williamson and Reginald Hems. Besides the technicians, two to three people were always working for their D.Phil. degrees in biochemistry. At 11 a.m., everyone gathered upstairs in a room for coffee and biscuits. Then all worked until lunch, which was eaten from a lunch bag, at Green College or at a nearby pub. All worked until 4 p.m. when we gathered for tea and biscuits. I found the tea gave me the stimulant I needed to finish up my work by 6 p.m., when we all went home.

We decided not to lease or purchase a car. Instead we went to a local bicycle shop and rented bikes, one for each of us. We learned to shop with our bikes and their attached baskets in nearby Summer Town or at the Closed Market in the center of Oxford. I rode to the lab in rain, snow, sleet or sunshine on my bicycle. Emily enrolled in the North Oxford comprehensive school, a city school but famous for its faculty and interesting mix of students from all classes of society and from many countries. She was placed in the sixth form (senior year) because the fifth-form students were studying for their O-level exams. She took courses in European History and American History taught from an English point of view. She also studied German and English literature. She was required to write essays every day. In addition to her schoolwork, she played flute in the school orchestra, took flute and math lessons and acted in plays. Her friends came to the door on Friday evenings in a group and took her out to pubs where they talked and drank hard cider and beer. She relaxed in the senior common room, went out to a bakery for lunch, gained weight on bakery sweets and swam at a nearby pool. I had never seen Emily so happy.

Marjorie was given a sabbatical leave for six months from the Indianapolis Public Schools because she agreed to research and write a paper on the education of the blind in England. We both obtained passes to admit us to the many Oxford libraries. She arranged day trips to cities where they had programs for the blind. She rode her bicycle to the train or bus station early in the morning and returned late to ride home in the dark with her bicycle lights on. She read books and papers on her subject in the Bodleian and education libraries. On weekends, I rented a small car and we made overnight visits to cities and cathedrals on the south coast, the city of Bath and the Cotswolds. I arranged by a generous donation to the crew coach at St. Edwards School to borrow single shells for Emily and me to row on the upper Thames River from their boathouse. Emily became a quite skilled sculler for a beginner.

In the lab, I tested assays of glutaminase in the mitochondria of rat livers and determined the kinetic constants for this enzyme. This was the first enzyme I had worked with that had an allosteric (S-shaped) activity response to increasing concentrations of its substrate glutamine. This was called positive cooperativity. Then I arranged with surgeons at the John Radcliffe Hospital to obtain informed consent from ten patients undergoing elective surgery for abdominal conditions. The surgeons were allowed to remove a one- to two-gram wedge biopsy of normal liver for my experiments. This offered little risk to these patients. I processed the biopsies by isolating their mitochondria and assaying glutamine cleavage by measuring glutamate or ammonia production. Our main findings were that the human liver glutaminase, like the rat liver enzyme, also showed positive cooperativity when exposed to glutamine and to phosphate, one of its activators. Ammonia also activated the human enzyme by reducing the glutamine concentration required to obtain half-maximal velocity of the reaction. Bicarbonate surprisingly did the same thing as ammonia. Human kidney glutaminase was a different enzyme. It showed a classical hyperbolic response to glutamine. It was inhibited by glutamate and had an absolute requirement for phosphate to be active. By July, I had finished writing my paper, which was published in 1984 in *Biochemica Biophysica Acta* and entitled "Allosteric Properties of Phosphate-Activated Glutaminase of Human Liver Mitochondria" by Snodgrass and Lund.

Once we were in Oxford, friends and relatives came to visit us. Over Easter holiday, Amy joined us and we flew to Munich to visit Martha. We rented a car and drove over the Brenner Pass into Italy. We went sightseeing in Verona, Florence, Sienna, Rome and Sorrento as well as other sites. A highlight was climbing Mt. Vesuvius, the girls wearing flip-flop sandals. We sat on rocks which turned out to harbor steam vents and gave the guide a good laugh as he caught another tourist with his favorite trick. Later in the summer Jennifer came over to join us on a trip to Wales and to the Lake District for hiking and horseback riding. Martha also visited us in Oxford. Amy stayed for two months and hiked the Lake District by herself. We learned how helpful the National Health System can be when Marjorie developed back trouble. An osteopathic physician treated her free of charge and recommended a physical therapist. Their treatment and exercises helped her resolve her back problem.

I was pleased to attend the yearly meeting of the British Gastroenterology Association with Derek Jewell, who was chief of the gastrointestinal section at Oxford. Reginald Strickland joined us on the trip. He was chief of gastroenterology at the University of New Mexico School of Medicine and was on a sabbatical leave in Derek's lab. Martin Sarner met us in Durham and introduced me to many famous British gastroenterologists. Sheila Sherlock, chief of medicine at the Royal Free Hospital, was most interested in my research and asked me to send my curriculum vitae. Later, she called and asked me to come to the Royal Free and give a lecture on Reye's syndrome, which was then occurring in Britain. At Oxford, I gave lectures on urea cycle enzyme induction and Reye's syndrome at the Radcliffe Infirmary. My friend and research colleague in Paris, Professor Liliane Cathelineau, and Daniel Rabier, her PhD colleague who worked a year in my lab in 1981, invited me to lecture at the Hôpital Enfants Malades, the children's hospital in Paris. They had seen more OTC deficiency and written more good clinical papers on the subject then I. However, my lecture on induction of the enzymes by hormones and amino acids was new to them. Although I had to speak in English, the lecture was understood and well received. Liliane then gave a dinner party for us at her rooftop apartment beginning with champagne at 6 p.m. and lasting through six courses until midnight. Finally, in May I was asked to lecture at the Hospital for Sick Children in London, where the research people were also experts in urea cycle deficiencies of all kinds. Again, our research on induction of the cycle was new and well received.

Emily had been chosen in Indianapolis to play the flute in a high school band called the American Musical Ambassadors, made up of top high school musicians across Indiana. She told them that when they took their summer tour of Europe, she would join them, coming from Oxford. The group landed in Paris and went by bus to a small town north of Amsterdam. Emily, by herself, flew to Amsterdam and took a train to this town, finally meeting up for rehearsals and a concert. One of the many cities where they performed was Innsbruck, Austria, where Martha came from Munich to hear them. When they performed in Paris, Marjorie and I showed up at the concert stage in Luxembourg Gardens. In London, we again attended their concert on the south bank of the Thames. Her bandmates were amazed by our family loyalty.

The MRL closed at the end of July and everyone went off on holiday. We spent the month traveling around England and flew back to Indianapolis by the first of September. When asked by a colleague at the medical school how I liked my sabbatical in Oxford, I said, "It was halfway to heaven."

13

Chief of the VA Medical Service and Professor of Medicine

✦

1983–1995

When I returned from Oxford in September 1982, I found the medical service had functioned well under the supervision of Dr. Ian Dowdeswell. My new chief resident, Jim Gaither, who had been chosen before I left on sabbatical, was functioning well and planning to go into pulmonary medicine. My laboratory progress however was disappointing. The experiments I had planned for one of my technicians came to no useful conclusions. Jeanine, who cared for the OTC mutant mouse colony, had mixed up their breeding status and allowed the mice to become infected with a *Chlamydia* bacterium. We had to restart the colony from newborns at Purdue and maintain sterile precautions in their feed and housing. Renee Lin and Catherine Maxey, my senior technician, made good progress in a study of rats whose adrenal glands were removed. The urea cycle enzymes could not be induced in these rats with glucagon, proving that as in cultured liver cells, the adrenal glucocorticoid hormones played a permissive role. Renee was now working on lipoproteins in cultured liver cells. It took two months for me to get the lab back on track again.

In 1981, Dean Steven Beering left to become president of Purdue University. A search committee chose Walter Daly as the new dean. He appointed August Watanabe, one of his former chief residents, and my chief of cardiology at the VA as interim chairmen. Dr. T.K. Li was chosen by Dean Daly to chair the search committee for a new chairperson of the Department of Medicine. I applied for the position of chairman as did Dr. Joseph Mamlin, the chief of the medical service at the Wishard (County) Hospital. Dr. Mamlin had been a faculty member longer than I and had created and developed the division of primary care medicine at the Wishard. This division recruited good internal medicine physicians from our program and elsewhere and staffed the outpatient clinics, emergency ward at the Wishard, two nursing homes, the new Geriatric program and later on the medicine clinics at the VA. He was Woody's personal physician and an excellent doctor in all respects.

T.K. Li contacted excellent academic people from the entire United States. At least six were invited for interviews before the search committee. Joe Mamlin and I were interviewed as well. My goals as stated to the committee were to elevate the department to be equal to the best in the Midwest, such as the University of Michigan and Washington University in St. Louis. I intended to devote myself full-time to teaching and to administration and planned to discontinue research because I knew that chairmen never had time to supervise their laboratories in the way they should. Dr. Daly declined to appoint each of the candidates interviewed, including Dr. Mamlin and myself. He finally decided to make the interim chairman, Dr August "Gus" Watanabe, the new chairman. I did not believe that my candidacy had ever been considered seriously.

Gus Watanabe and I worked well enough together. I brought up again to him the fact that in most academic VA hospitals the chief of medical service's salary was supplemented by the department of medicine. Dr. Watanabe told me that he would not supplement my VA salary even though it was now well below that of full professors of medicine at the University Hospital. Gus said that if I needed to increase my salary, I would have to earn it by working in the Gastrointestinal Clinic at the University Hospital.

I was asked to be a visiting professor at the University of Wisconsin Medical School in Madison, my hometown. There I gave a grand rounds lecture on urea cycle induction. The former dean, William Middleton, congratulated me on the presentation and asked where I had attended medical school since I said I had graduated from Madison West High School. I told him that after he turned me down for admission to the University of Wisconsin Medical School, I had to take my second choice, Harvard. He looked distressed and apologized for turning me down but obviously did not remember the interview with him in 1948. In 1983, I was also invited to be a visiting professor at the University of Texas in San Antonio and gave grand rounds on the urea cycle. After these happy experiences, I decided to find a position as chairman of medicine at another U.S. medical school. I was contacted by medical schools in Hawaii, Wisconsin and North Carolina who were searching for new chairpersons in medicine. I submitted my curriculum vitae to Wisconsin and North Carolina and asked George Thorn and Walter Daly to write letters of support. I never knew what Dr. Thorn said, but I heard that Dr. Daly wrote a curt letter saying, "If he wants the job, he can do it," I never was asked to appear for an interview at either medical school.

It became apparent to me that Dean Daly and Gus Watanabe did not want me to leave the VA, where I was doing an excellent job for them. When we had visits from the Joint Commission on Accreditation of Healthcare Organizations at the VA, Dean Daly told me that it was my job to see that the VA passed inspection, even though it was the surgery and radiology services that were having problems meeting the requirements. I helped coach them through the paperwork and did most of the hospital presentation before the committee, describing our successful program of continuing quality improvement.

As chief of the VA, I had previously offered the chief residency to three different female senior residents. They turned me down, stating that the staff, nurses and employees on the medical service would not welcome a female chief resident. In 1983, I asked Debra Helper to be my chief resident and she accepted. She said that she was not concerned about the male-oriented culture at the VA. Debra was the daughter of a professor at the University of Illinois. She attended Indiana University for college and Northwestern University for medical school, excelling at both places. As an intern and resident, she had been outstanding and a leader. As my chief resident, she made a number of suggestions to improve the service. Instead of holding morning report every morning as we did at the Brigham, she wanted to have one morning free for the discussion of a case selected from the wards of the hospital. She and I chose a staff person from the faculty to monitor the discussion and make recommendations on diagnosis and management. Dr. Dowdeswell and I always attended these presentations. The house staff and students warmly welcomed these teaching sessions.

During the year, Debra discussed possible career choices in academic medicine and settled on gastroenterology. She began a fellowship doing basic research on the smooth muscle of the esophageal sphincter and her abstract after six month's work was chosen for oral presentation at the gastrointestinal meetings in Chicago. Unfortunately her research mentor left the faculty and she lost interest in laboratory research. She took time out to have a baby boy and then finished her clinical gastrointestinal training, had another baby boy and then became the director of the Indiana gastroenterology program on inflammatory bowel disease. She became an acknowledged expert in this area and was promoted to clinical professor of medicine.

The rest of my subsequent chief residents were again male. E. Randolph Broun developed ulcerative colitis during residency training but I offered him the chief residency in spite of the risk. He stayed well and did well and trained in hematology later, ending up as a professor at St. Louis University. In 1986–1987 Tom Ryan helped Ian Dowdeswell reorganize the coronary care and intensive care unit rotations, a project Ian had been working on for two years. Previously, each team from the ward and their attending physician admitted and cared for patients on these units, supervised by a cardiology staff in the Coronary Care Unit and a pulmonary staff in the Intensive Care Unit. Ian convinced me and Tom agreed that we needed a separate intensive care rotation for interns and residents staffed full-time by cardiologists and pulmonary specialists. Then the nurses would not have to deal with eight different teams of house staff and attendings who might be weak in intensive care management. The new rotation was a huge success with the residents, nurses and pulmonary technicians. Tom Ryan trained in cardiology, became an expert in cardiac ultrasound and later went to Duke University as an assistant professor. I cannot detail the names, accomplishments, and subsequent careers of the eight chief residents from 1987 to 1995. Suffice it to say that all went on to specialize in some area of internal medicine and all but three went into practice. These three chose to stay in academic medicine.

In 1987, I asked the VA to predict what my civil service retirement income would be in 1995, when I planned to retire at age 67. I was shocked to hear that it would be roughly $40,000 per year if my high three salary years increased as expected. This would not be adequate for a decent retirement for Marjorie and me. I had a small amount in TIAA-CREF from my days at Harvard, but it had grown slowly and no additional money had gone into the account because Indiana University School of Medicine never paid me any salary. I asked my friend and colleague, Dr. Larry Lumeng, now the chief of gastroenterology in the Department of Medicine, if I could work one day a week in the gastrointestinal clinic at University Hospital. I was taking Gus Watanabe's advice to earn my supplement. Larry agreed to pay me $12,000 a year but would expect that my collections in the clinic would pay for this plus the administrative costs that I incurred. So I rearranged my full-time VA schedule to allow me to work Wednesdays from 10 a.m. to 6 p.m. in the clinic. My appointments were booked solid every clinic day and I found myself seeing mostly women with similar problems to those I had seen in private practice back at the Brigham. The gastrointestinal staff sent me patients who were not going to require endoscopy procedures, which is where the division derived most of its income. I was doing no procedures. I usually saw women with chronic abdominal pain, constipation or diarrhea and rarely saw patients with liver or pancreatic diseases, where I excelled. All of the after-tax income I was paid went into my TIAA-CREF account. The economic boom in the 1990s helped this account grow rapidly and salvaged my retirement problems.

The VA Research Service in Central Office in Washington, D.C. asked me to be an advisor and member of review groups from 1977 through 1988. I chaired site visits to research services at many VA hospitals, doing my best to help them improve their programs. This allowed me to meet again former students, residents and colleagues, a most enjoyable benefit. The review of individual investigators by our committee was quite stressful. During one interview at the Manhattan VA, a man developed a myocardial infarction (heart attack) while sitting at the table.

I was chosen to sit on various planning committees at Central Office and became acquainted with the best directors, chiefs of staff and chiefs of service in the VA system. In 1986 I became a member of the Merit Review Board in gastroenterology, which reviewed, approved or disapproved and recommended funding for the gastrointestinal research grant applications throughout the VA system. I took a leadership role in the committee and actually read, took notes on and asked questions about the 40 to 60 grants we reviewed three times a year. In 1988, I was chosen as chairman of this merit review board. My reviews and decisions were rigorous but fair. I actually helped boost gastrointestinal funding above other merit review boards and other specialties. My own research funding by NIH on urea cycle induction ceased in 1980 because the topics were considered too similar to my ongoing VA grants.

One of the most stressful experiences in academic medicine was writing grant applications and renewal applications. The usual funding was for three years. It took a whole year to review past accomplishments and then present new ideas for studies which would be seen as "cutting edge" by the review board. My experience on VA review boards helped but the VA basic science merit review board, which reviewed my grants, was the most difficult to please. I developed a system for keeping up with urea cycle and ammonia biochemistry by reading *Chemical Abstracts* and photocopying the pertinent articles in the library. Eventually this could be done on a computer using search engines like Pub Med from the Library of Congress. If a renewal was judged borderline, it needed to be rewritten and resubmitted. Fortunately, I always came in with a score in the safe funding zone through 1993. The jobs of my technicians and my PhD depended on the success of these grant renewal applications. I felt a great responsibility toward all of them. I saw doctors at our VA turned down as nonfundable even after they had reapplied. It was a devastating blow to these investigators' self-esteem. Some just quit research and moved to the University Hospital to do clinical work or went into private practice. The fault lay mostly in our training system. A graduating senior resident would join a specialty research division and be placed in the laboratory, where he was taught some research techniques but not how to go about designing, carrying out and writing up a research project. Then he was helped to write a grant application and had an even chance of getting funding. If he was funded, alone in his own laboratory with one technician he rarely accomplished enough to deserve a renewal of his grant. Mentoring by experienced and successful investigators was often lacking. These young people quit research after two to three years and left to go into private practice. What a waste of young talent and a loss for academic medicine!

I published papers in the *Journal of Nutrition* in 1987, in *Hepatology* in 1989 and in *Enzyme* in 1991, all concerned with urea cycle induction and various model systems. I continued to collaborate with other investigators to study OTC deficiency in their patients. In 1989, Renee Lin asked to leave the laboratory and join Dr. Larry Lumeng in his studies of alcohol metabolism and alcohol-preferring rats. Her independent research had not been very successful. Her grant was canceled and she was no longer interested in doing urea cycle work. She and I parted on the best of terms and remained friends and colleagues. With success in Dr. Lumeng's laboratory, she was promoted to full professor on the research track in the Department of Medicine, which was her lifelong goal.

I was fortunate to find a new PhD, Corrine Ulbright, who had some experience in molecular biology and DNA and RNA research. These were the very topics toward which I was planning to move my research. Corrine obtained from other investigators complementary DNAs (cDNAs) for each of the urea cycle enzymes. Thus, we could measure messenger RNA levels and rates of mRNA synthesis (nuclear transcription). She became expert in all the technical details of isolating total RNA from cultured rat liver cells, labeling the cDNAs with radioactive nucleotides, separating the RNAs by electrophoresis, making autoradiographs of the radiolabeled mRNA bands and measuring their amounts by scanning the radiographs. This was all beyond my experience and I watched the procedures in awe. We compared stable mRNA levels, nuclear transcription rates, and enzyme activities after induction by glucagon and dexamethasone, a potent synthetic adrenal glucocorticoid. The increase in all five enzyme activities was accomplished by three different mechanisms in the DNA-RNA-protein sequence. This important manuscript, a capstone to our work on urea cycle induction for thirty-five years, was published in the *Archives of Biochemistry and Biophysics* in 1993. Corrine and I then decided that we could go no farther in the molecular biology of urea cycle induction with only an MD, a PhD and two technicians. To analyze the control of gene activation at what were called promoter and enhancer regions of the DNA on the five genes was beyond our capability, so we would leave such work to large molecular biology laboratories that did this kind of research routinely. Thus, I decided to close my laboratory in 1993 and said goodbye to Corrine and my last technicians. Catherine and Bill, my original technicians, had retired and others had gone on to better jobs with Eli Lilly Company or at the medical school. I sent my colony of OTC deficient mice to the group at Baylor University School of Medicine, who made good use of them in their research. I never did make any important new findings using this animal model.

After careful consideration, I decided to write a book about OTC covering all the clinical and basic science knowledge about this key enzyme in the urea cycle. I began to collect everything in the world literature about this enzyme and dictated a number of first draft chapters, which my efficient secretary, Carol Mechuta, typed for me. My retirement day was July 15, 1995, determined by the end of the last eight-year extension of my VA contract. The VA gave me a reception where all my friends, former employees and present VA staff could say goodbye.

My executive assistant, Michael Goodelle, and my wife planned in secret an extravagant farewell party at the University Place Hotel. Dr. Craig Brater, the new chairman of medicine, paid for the hall, food and band. I was surprised to have my three daughters from Boston, my sister and her husband from Dallas, and Marjorie's two cousins from California show up on a Friday. We drove to the hotel ostensibly to have dinner together and there were all my friends and colleagues gathered in the ballroom for a banquet, speeches and dancing. T.K. Li presented my early life from childhood through the Boston years with humor and gentle ribbing. Ian Dowdeswell was master of ceremonies for the Indianapolis years. So many people wanted to toast or roast old Dr. Snodgrass that no time was left for dancing. At least ten of my chief residents showed up and all wanted to tell stories about their year with me. Afterward, many people said it was the best retirement party they had ever attended. This was all due to the planning and efforts of my wife, Marjorie, and Mike Goodelle, my last and best office administrator. Two days later, Marjorie and I left for a month's vacation at our favorite place in Maine, the Five Kezar Ponds, where we first stayed in 1958. For me, my career in the Veteran's Administration came to a close with a sense of great personal satisfaction. In retrospect I realize that my leaving Harvard and the Brigham hospital for Indiana University School of Medicine and the VA hospital was the best outcome for my career and happiness in academic medicine. Every morning when I awoke in Indianapolis I looked forward to going to work at the VA hospital!

14

Retirement

When I returned from vacation in Maine, I was told of a tragedy which had occurred at the Roudebush VA Medical Center shortly after I left. Our new director, a woman, had been there six months and had caused me and the other service chiefs few problems. After I left, she called a meeting of the psychiatry service and in front of the doctors and nurses and other staff people she demoted to a staff position our chief of the psychiatry service, John Sullivan. Jack, as we called him, came to us from Central Office Psychiatry Service. He had been trained at Johns Hopkins Medical School and Hospital as an internist and then went into psychiatry. He had been at our hospital about four years and was well liked by the hospital staff and the people at the IU School of Medicine. I worked with him on committees and found him to be intelligent and able. Apparently, he was a poor administrator in the opinion of our new director. She wanted to appoint a new chief of psychiatry but did not discuss her plans with Jack privately. When she announced the change in front of his entire psychiatry staff, she told Jack that he could stay on as a staff psychiatrist or go somewhere else. Three days later Jack committed suicide with a bullet to the head. We did not know that Jack had been having emotional problems. He was divorced before he came to Indianapolis and had been depressed on and off but he kept it well hidden behind his usual affability and good humor. This suicide caused a scandal in Indianapolis, our hospital, the medical school and in the Central Office in Washington. Our director was reassigned to a regional office. Ian Dowdeswell, my assistant chief of medicine, told me that after this episode morale plummeted and has only slowly recovered.

I changed my private clinic to Monday afternoons and continued to see general gastroenterology patients, doing my customary one-hour work-ups for new patients. I attended medical grand rounds every Wednesday morning as usual and tried to ask a pertinent question no matter what the topic. Then I worked in the medical library, searching the literature for old and new articles on ornithine transcarbamylase and the urea cycle and photocopying articles for the writing of my book on OTC.

In September 1995, I was preparing to go to Eldoret, Kenya, as a one-month visiting professor at the Moi Medical School, with which Indiana University School of Medicine had developed a partnership. Joseph Mamlin, chief of medicine at the Wishard Hospital, had always been involved in international medicine. He had established a partnership with a medical school in Kabul, Afghanistan, but it was destroyed by the Soviet invasion and later civil war. He and Robert Einterz, my personal physician, searched around the world to find a country and medical school with which to associate. They chose Kenya and Moi Medical School, named after the president of Kenya, who came from the city of Eldoret in Northwest Kenya, near the border with Uganda. This high plateau was fertile and less plagued by malaria than the lowlands. The Moi University had just opened and the Moi Medical School was only a single building and an old district hospital from British colonial days. Joe Mamlin offered to base an Indiana faculty member and family for one-year terms in Eldoret. They would live in a large house behind a walled compound, which we called Indiana House, and host other volunteers from our medical school. Other Indiana University School of Medicine faculty volunteered to spend one to two months there to work with the Dean of Moi Medical School and his three faculty members. We shared in teaching the twenty Moi Medical students basic science and clinical medicine and helped the Kenyans care for patients on the wards of the hospital. We began to rotate residents from our Indiana house staff for one- to two-month terms in the hospital, and our medical students began to elect a one- to two-month experience there as well. By 1995, we had been there six years. Joe and his wife spent the first year. Bob Einterz and his family spent the second year, and four other members of Joe's internal medicine faculty each spent a year there with their families. Before we left for our month of service, Marjorie and I were given 22 inoculations or oral vaccines for most of the diseases we would encounter there, except for malaria. There is no vaccine for malaria. All Americans took weekly doses of various drugs to prevent the resistant and dangerous *Falciparum* malaria, which is endemic in Kenya.

I had been training and competing in single-shell races all summer and had been accepted by lottery to row in the Head of the Charles Regatta in Boston on October 17th. We planned to leave for Kenya a few days later. I left the Cambridge Boat Club dock to cross from the Cambridge to the Boston side of the Charles River in order to go down to the starting line three miles below. I thought there was a safe gap between the women's four-oared shells which were racing upriver. As I crossed over, a boat with a crew of four women and coxswain from the Lake Washington Rowing Club came rapidly around the corner and their bow stuck me in the right calf, throwing me into the water. My boat amazingly was not damaged. As I turned to swim the boat to shore, intending to climb back in and row the race, I felt severe pain in my right calf and saw that the river was turning red with my blood behind me. I called for help and a woman rower from Middlebury College who had finished the race dove in the water and helped me and my boat to get to shore. There, a woman doctor came to my help and put a tourniquet around my thigh to stop the bleeding. The emergency medical technicians took me to Mount Auburn Hospital Emergency Ward, where I was hypothermic and had a low blood pressure. The original X-ray showed no broken bones. I only had minor loss of feeling in the right foot, but luckily no serious nerve injury After they gave me intravenous fluids, I came around somewhat and a woman resident then spent three hours sewing up my torn calf muscles, the covering layers called "fascia" and the skin. They then sent me to my daughter Jennifer's apartment in Cambridge, and a day later when I came back to the emergency ward for a check-up, my packed red blood cell volume had fallen from its normal of 44% to 22%. In other words, I had lost half my red cell volume in the Charles River. Partly to blame was the fact that I took 81 mg of aspirin everyday, which prevented my platelets from clotting my blood. Because the surgeon left no drain in the wound, the severed muscle arteries bled into my calf and down into my foot, causing the whole lower leg to swell up with a great blue-red hematoma. Luckily, I did not develop blood clots in the leg veins, which could have gone to my lungs. We flew home and I recovered for three weeks. Then we flew to Kenya.

Coming late, I saw the students only two weeks before they left on Christmas holiday. I did give a grand rounds talk about hepatitis C, which was just being recognized as a major illness throughout Africa. Dr. Kimayo, the Kenya internist with whom I made rounds each day, taught me more about African medicine than I taught him about American medicine and gastroenterology. At the time, we had no surgical or pathology services, inadequate X-ray and laboratory services, and a constant shortage of basic medications. Only five antibiotics were available and we often supplied them from our stock in Indiana House when the pharmacy ran out. I had no Indiana resident physician on my male ward of 50 patients (two to a bed), no Kenya intern and only a male nurse practitioner and the ward nurses. They were experts in treating malarial coma with intravenous quinine and diabetic coma with insulin. The patients spoke many village dialects and little Swahili, which I was just learning, so we could not get good histories.

Physical examination was the only diagnostic tool. I missed a case of flagrant pellagra in a man with dermatitis, dementia and diarrhea. This disorder is due to a deficiency of the B-vitamin niacin. Dr. Kimayo recognized it immediately. I did diagnose a man with a brain abscess, confirmed by reading my own crude electroencephalogram but, no neurosurgeon was available to drain it. We gave him various antibiotics but eventually he died. I saw fatal tetanus in a boy of 12 who had been circumcised by a village doctor using a dirty stone knife. I watched an 8-year-old boy die with acute glomerulonephritis (post-streptococcal inflammation) and total renal failure. We could not get his kidneys to work with diuretics and he drowned in his own lung fluids.

In mid-December, all the Indiana people went on vacation or went home. Dr. Kimayo was so busy with private patients he could only visit one day a week. I was left to care for 50 severely ill patients. We had 5 to 10 new admissions every day and no support system. I did my best, guessing at what diseases they might have and treating them with the antibiotics I had, but many people died. The prevalence of HIV infection was recognized by a fungal growth in the mouth which is a sign of late AIDS. We did have a screening test for HIV and I found that 30% of our patients carried the virus. We treated their lung lesions which we saw on X-ray with trimethoprim-sulfa if we thought it was *Pneumocystis* superinfection. If it looked like tuberculosis we gave them streptomycin and isoniazid.

Marjorie and I lived alone in a separate house down the hill from Indiana House. In the main house we cooked our own meals after the cook left on vacation. Marjorie volunteered at the Testimony Faith Home and School, a place for orphan children. Most were boys because girls are valuable and do most of the work in Kenya. Many of the boys lived on the town dump scavenging for food. If they were lucky, Mr. and Mrs. Green brought them to the school where they were fed, clothed, educated and loved. The unlucky boys lived briefly in a shelter called the Rescue Mission. We went there weekly to examine and prescribe for them. The 13-year-olds were only the size of 8-year-old boys and were covered with skin diseases.

On weekends, Dr. Robert Bond, the professor who was living there with his family, drove us and his family to lodges on lakes in the Rift Valley or to the Kakamega Rain Forrest. These were our first views of African village life and of African wildlife. When the staff returned from their holiday after the first of January, Marjorie and I went on a ten-day bird-watching safari, led by a marvelous Kenyan guide. We saw about 400 species of birds and almost every Kenyan animal as we drove over the country, from the mountains to the deserts and to the Masai Mara, the Great Plains of Kenya. As we left, I felt so sad, frustrated and angry that I could not do more for these wonderful patients. Kenyans we met were so bright and friendly and welcoming to Americans.

In the next ten years, amazing progress was made. A surgical pavilion was built. A surgeon spent five years there and others followed. Pathology and laboratory services were improved. A pediatric intensive care unit and an obstetrical unit were set up. Kenyan doctors came to train in Indianapolis. A number of U.S. medical schools joined the program as a part of a consortium. Finally, a pilot study for the treatment of HIV was begun using modern drug regimens, supervised by Kenyan doctors and trained native women in village clinics. Their compliance rate was 90 percent for taking their medicines. The Moi students came to Indianapolis for two months to see American medicine at the Wishard Hospital. One of the problems was the lack of good practice positions in Kenya or Africa after our Moi students graduated.

When I returned from Kenya, I went to work seriously on my OTC book. First I had to learn to type. This was accomplished by working with a computerized teaching system. Eventually, I was able to type 15 words per minute with roughly 10% errors. From 1996 to 2000, I was able to complete 9 chapters, containing 700 references. Jennifer, my second daughter and an editor at Harvard University Press, put me in touch with an editor at Kluwer Academic Publishers. After listening to my description of the book, she asked me to send a finished chapter and a plan for the other chapters for her to review. I sent her the completed manuscript and the review board agreed to publish it. They insisted that I update all chapters throughout 2002, which forced me to rewrite most of the chapters. Finally, it was accepted. I had to pay a firm to do the electronic typesetting, including all the tables and figures. Finally, Kluwer came through and produced a beautiful hardcover book on high-grade paper. I designed a cover which showed the title, *Ornithine Transcarbamylase*, at the top in a balloon with a tail entering a schematic cell and mitochondrion. There the urea cycle was shown in terms of its substrates like ammonia and products such as ornithine, citrulline and arginine. The point of the tail pointed directly to the OTC reaction where ornithine was changed into citrulline. The subtitle of the book was "Basic Science and Clinical Considerations." Surprisingly, Kluwer agreed to use this unusual cover design.

One thousand copies were printed and I sent complimentary books to the people who helped me review and advised me about the book. Then I sent advertising brochures and personal notes to 100 investigators around the world whom I knew were interested in OTC and the urea cycle. I received many complimentary letters, usually commenting that they were impressed that I undertook to write this book by myself. Most scientific books are done by a group of chapter authors and edited by one or two other people. Fortunately, the burst of knowledge and understanding about the urea cycle and OTC from 1962 to 2002 had reached a plateau. Publications since then have added only details. The book accomplished what I intended: to sum up in one volume everything that is known about this important enzyme, its 3-dimensional structure, DNA and protein sequences, genetics, animal models, clinical deficiencies, and treatment of the affected patients. The last chapter summarized our work and those of others on the induction and suppression of the urea cycle, especially OTC. It described the mechanisms of gene control of the five enzymes. Only those interested in the urea cycle will read this book but they will find an analysis of the research literature and the references needed to pursue their own work, be it basic science or clinical care.

While I was writing my book, Marjorie was writing two books. One was an oral history of students and teachers during the first fifty years of Arsenal Technical High School. She and her brother had graduated there, and her mother taught there and met her father there. He taught German and Spanish for forty years at that school. It was a popular book, self-published, that sold all 1000 copies printed. Her second book was an oral history of the students she taught at Perkins School for the Blind in Watertown Massachusetts. The students had been in her first-grade classes from 1950 to 1954. When she interviewed them they were in their 50s. The book gave poignant insights into the lives of blind children and their subsequent careers.

I ceased seeing clinic patients in June of 1999 and became professor emeritus from Indiana University School of Medicine. Since then, I have continued rowing competitively. The most recent big race was the Head of the Charles Regatta in 2004. I started last, 26th among the senior veterans (over 70), and finished 21st. I continue to read the main medical journals because I am a confirmed biology and medicine watcher. I review the urea cycle literature on my computer search system for the same reason.

My last experience as a practicing physician occurred at my wife's 55th Reunion at Oberlin College. A classmate collapsed in his chair in the lounge after dinner and none of the other doctors stepped forward. I pulled him from his chair to the floor, laid him on his back and found no pulse. A classmate's wife who had been a nurse helped me bare his chest, where I noted large scars. His wife then told me that he had had two cardiac bypass operations in the past ten years and had severely impaired heart function. I began immediate cardiac compression. We did not have to give him mouth-to-mouth respiration because he began to breathe on his own. After 15 minutes, the firemen arrived, hooked up an EKG and found, as I guessed, that he was in ventricular fibrillation, an arrhythmia where the heart quivers but does not contract. We hooked up a defibrillator and shocked him three times before we got him into a functional rhythm and felt a pulse. He awoke and spoke as they carried him out to the local hospital. He kept going back into fibrillation and they gave him at least 20 defibrillation shocks as they transferred him to the Elyria (Ohio) Heart Center. By the next morning, to my amazement he was awake and able to talk and eat a regular meal. A permanent defibrillator was installed in his heart and then he went back to his hometown near Cincinnati. I spoke to him and his wife on the phone and he was doing well with no episodes of defibrillator discharges. Sadly, his wife called three months later and said that he had died suddenly. His last three months were full of joy and family visits. This was the first person upon whom I had performed cardiopulmonary resuscitation alone since I was a resident at the Brigham. The old training had just kicked in and I did it properly. Rarely had I ever had a success like this one. Hopefully I will not have to do resuscitation again on anyone because I cannot expect such a good outcome.

Thus, I conclude my memoir. Marjorie and I have moved from Indianapolis to Peabody, Massachusetts, to a retirement village to be near three of our four daughters. What a wonderful life I have had in academic medicine over these years from 1953 to 2005. My gratitude goes out to all the wonderful patients, colleagues, doctors, nurses, and others for their part in enriching my life.

Index

Abbruzzese, Americo 90, **101**, 102, 106, 121
Adelstein, S. James 29, **76**
Aesculapian Club 26
Albright, Fuller 16, 24

Babior, Bernard M. 75
Beering, Steven C. 121, **133**, 139
Blattner, Russell J. 53
Boston Lying-in Hospital 10, 20, 35, 36, 52, 54, 57, 59, 77
Bradley, Dorothy 117
Braunwald, Eugene 115
Brooks, John R. 16, **93**, 102
Buchner, David M. 125
Burwell, C. Sidney 40, 44

Cahill, George F., Jr. 29
Cathelineau, Liliane 138
Chang, Lennig 109, **110**
Chinook salmon 105, 106
Coley, Geoffrey M. 9
Curtis, Stephen J. 102, **103**

Daly, Walter J. 115, 117, 120, 121, 122, 125, 127, 130, **133**, 139, 140
Denny-Brown, Derek 18
DES, diethylstilbestrol 54
Dieckman, Merwin 50, 53
Doll, Sir W. Richard S. 92, **135**
Dowdeswell, Ian 130, **134**, 139, 142, 145, 147
Dye, Eugene N. 2, 4, 17, 18

Earle, A. Scott 14, 17
Eisenlohr, John E. 50, 51, 53, 86
Eppinger, Eugene C. 35, 41, 56, 80, 84, **87**, 116
Epstein, Charles J. 75, 78

Finch, Clement A. 8, 41
Foley, Joseph M. 63, 64
Fuglestad, Vercel 50, 53

Glutaminase, human liver 134, **137**
Goldberg, Morton F. 84, **85**
Gore, Ira 74
Gorlin, Richard 33
Gray, David H. 9, **27**
Gray, Seymour J. 89, **90**

Halothane 95
Halver, John E. 105, **106**
Hansen, Frederik C. 9, **15**
Harken, Dwight D. 60
Harold Amos 9, 81
Harrison's Textbook of Medicine 99, 100
Harter, John G. 29, 62
Harvard College 4, 5, 6, 8, 9, 12, 22, 23, 27, 84, 86, 125
Harvard Medical School ix, 7, 8, 9, 12, 21, 23, 29, 36, 54, 56, 76, 82, 83, 84, 86, 91, 99, 102, 106, 107, 112, 115, 116
Helper, Debra 141
Himmelhoch, S. Ralph 80, **83**
Hoch, Frederic L. 71
Hoerr, Robert A. 125

155

Holder, Richmond 18, 23
Hoover, Robert 50

Indiana University School of Medicine. 152
Ingelfinger, Franz J. 64, 92, 99, 100
Ireland, Patricia 109
Isselbacher, Kurt J. 91, 92, 101, 115

Jeffrey, Russell L. 96, 111
Joslin Clinic 64, 65, 105
Joslin Elliott P. 64, 65

Kaegi, Jeremias H. R. 71
Khaja, Nazir-uddin 112
Kingsville N.A.A.S. 43, 44
Krebs, Sir Hans A. 133

Levine, Samuel A. 38, 40, 76, 99
Liebowitz, Martin R, 56, 76
Lin, Renee C. 122, 134, 139, 144
Littmann, David 73
Li, Ting Kai 75, 115, 119
Lown, Bernard 38, 59, 106
Lumeng, Lawrence 120
Lund, Patricia 134

Mamlin, Joseph 139, 148
Maxey, Catherine 118, 126, 139
McKittrick, Leland S. 26
Metabolic Research Laboratory 133, 134, 135
Metcalfe, James 59
Middleton, William S. 7
Moore, Francis D. 31, 76
Moore, Merrill 22, 23
Moritz, Mordekhai 102, 104
Murphy, William P. 39
Murray, Joseph E. 16, 41

Nuzum, C. Thomas 97, 113, 114, 124

Oberlin College 11, 54, 119, 130, 152
Ornithine transcarbamylase 96, 103, 123, 126, 148, 151
Oxford University, England 134, 135
O'Hare, J. P. 40

Parry, David J. 96, 97
Perkins School for the Blind 20, 21, 35, 107, 152
Peter Bent Brigham Hospital ix, 8, 15, 17, 20, 29, 30, 31, 38, 55, 56, 73, 80, 90, 109
Peters, James I., Jr. 11, 12
Peters, John 117
Poliomyelitis 52

Q fever 51, 55

Rayyes, Amer 112, 113
Renold, Albert E. 29
Reye's syndrome 123, 124, 138
Robin, Eugene D. 29, 35

Sarner, Martin 102, 112, 132
Snodgrass, Marjorie (Woody) 11, 12, 13, 14, 17, 20, 45, 54, 70, 119, 136, 152
   Amy 77, 119, 131, 137
   Emily 104, 105, 119, 131, 132, 135, 136, 137, 138
   Jennifer 58, 69, 119, 131, 137, 149, 151
   Martha 46, 53, 54, 130, 137, 138

Thiers, Ralph 67, 68
Thomas, E. Donnall 8, 16, 41
Thorn, George W. 19, 25, 31, 76, 88, 100

Ulbright, Corrine 144
Urea cycle enzymes 95, 97, 98, 101, 111, 114, 123, 126, 127, 139, 144

U.S. Forest Service
  Clearwater National Forest, Idaho 11

Vallee Bert L. 65, 67, 72
Veterans Administration Hospitals
  R.L.Roudebush, Indianapolis, Indiana 128
  West Roxbury, Mass. 60

Wacker, Warren E. C. 32, 65, 69, 75, 78, 80, 106, 111, 115, 116
Walling, Heywood 46
Warthin, Thomas A. 60, 74
Watanabe, August M. 139
Weiner, Stanley 43
Weinstein, Louis 64, 74
Whitcomb, John H. 9, 11, 15
Wolf, Marshall 86
Wunsch, Sabine 131

978-0-595-44253-9
0-595-44253-6